STAYING
SAFE
Backyard to
Backcountry

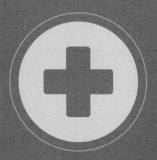

Patrick Brighton, MD

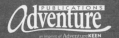

PUBLICATIONS
adventure
an imprint of AdventureKEEN

*This work is dedicated to the most complete person
I have ever known. To my adventure partner,
my best friend, my love, and my wife.
Thank you, Kimberley.*

Cover design: Travis Bryant and Jonathan Norberg

Interior design: Jonathan Norberg

Editors: Brett Ortler, Emily Beaumont, and Jenna Barron

Proofreader: Holly Cross

Indexer: Potomac Indexing

Library of Congress Cataloging-in-Publication Data

Names: Brighton, Patrick, 1962- author.

Title: Staying safe : backyard to backcountry / Patrick Brighton, M.D., FACS.

Identifiers: LCCN 2023016063 (print) | LCCN 2023016064 (ebook) | ISBN 9781647552794 (paperback) | ISBN 9781647553906 (ebook)

Subjects: LCSH: First aid in illness and injury--Popular works. | Wounds and injuries--Treatment--Popular works. | Medical emergencies--Popular works.

Classification: LCC RC87 .B783 2023 (print) | LCC RC87 (ebook) | DDC 616.02/52--dc23/eng/20230722

10 9 8 7 6 5 4 3 2 1

Staying Safe: Backyard to Backcountry
Copyright © 2023 by Patrick Brighton
Adventure Publications
An imprint of AdventureKEEN
310 Garfield Street South
Cambridge, MN 55008
(800) 678-7006
www.adventurepublications.net
ISBN 978-1-64755-279-4 (pbk.); ISBN 978-1-64755-390-6 (ebook)

TABLE OF CONTENTS

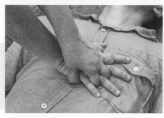

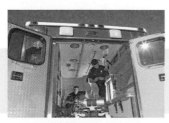

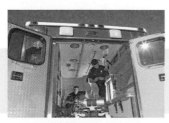

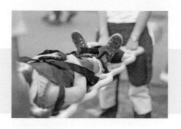

FIRST THINGS FIRST: AIRWAY, BREATHING, CIRCULATION, AND CPR

Medical terminology includes an almost limitless quantity of confusing and unnecessary acronyms. These will generally be avoided in this text except when special emphasis is required. This chapter represents one of those occasions. Life-threatening emergency situations require immediate action, and in such cases, a simple acronym can help you remember exactly what to do.

When individuals are faced with a medical emergency, whether it's a traumatic event injury or the result of a medical condition, the natural human response is dismay and even terror. But such feelings, however natural, can prevent first responders from providing prompt lifesaving care.

That's where the mnemonic **ABC** comes in: **Airway, Breathing, Circulation.** Brief and easy to follow, the ABCs help calm rescuers and tell them precisely where to start, as well as the sequence of subsequent steps. We'll cover the ABCs below.

A—Airway   B—Breathing   C—Circulation

Why ABC? Fortunately, these letters represent the beginning of the alphabet that we all learned as toddlers, and thus they are ingrained into our subconscious, but they also represent the sequence of bodily systems that, when they fail, will kill us in descending order of rapidity.

The airway is nothing more than a hollow tube that allows for free passage of inhaled air (including oxygen) and expired waste gases (including carbon dioxide). For our purposes, the limits of the airway include the nasal passages (nares) and lips (upper extent of the airway) to the vocal cords. The vocal cords are two flaps of tissue that separate the upper airway from the lower airway. They reside inside the trachea, roughly at the level of the Adam's apple. Although the airway technically extends to the very outer fringes of the lungs (alveoli), we describe the airway in these

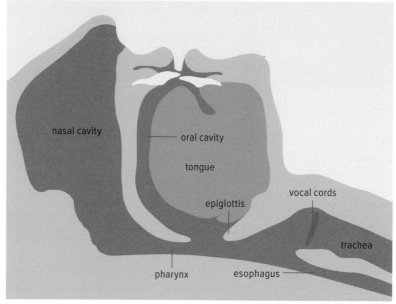

A simplified drawing of the human airway

terms because this section represents the only portion that nonadvanced medical responders may be able to clear in the event of an obstruction.

STEP 1: AIRWAY

No matter whether someone appears to be having a seizure, heart attack, or some other medical ailment—or if they have sustained severe bodily trauma, especially to the head or face—airway assessment should be the first and only initial consideration for a rescuer. The patient may be gasping for air, spitting up blood or vomit, or unconscious. Regardless, the airway needs to be investigated and cleared completely before any other assessment or treatment is undertaken. The sequence for this is as follows:

With the patient on the ground and turned slightly

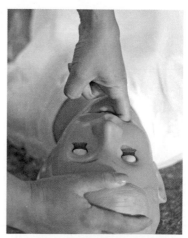

The proper technique for sweeping out the airway

onto one side, the rescuer (with gloved hands and eye protection if possible) opens the victim's mouth in a scissoring motion with the thumb and middle finger of the nondominant hand. With the dominant hand, the rescuer then sweeps from side-to-side to expel any foreign objects such as blood, bone, or foreign material. Since most humans are right-handed, it is typically easier to place the victim on their right side between 45–90 degrees—the rescue position. The rescuer should kneel above the head of the patient to achieve maximum access and leverage capabilities.

Only after the airway is open (patent in medical terminology) does the rescuer proceed with assessing the breathing status of the patient. Clearing the airway should take no more than a few seconds in most cases, so assessing if/how a patient is breathing as a second priority should not be detrimental.

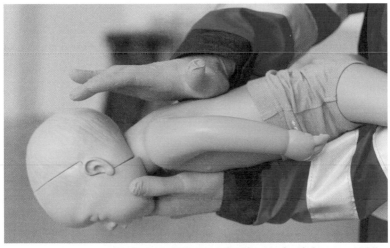

How to manually clear the airway of an infant or a toddler

If an infant's or small toddler's airway cannot be cleared manually, a child can be held upside-down while a sharp blow is delivered between the shoulder blades to dislodge any foreign body from an impacted airway.

What happens if we can't clear the airway? If there is an obstruction farther down the passageway and we are unable to extract it, the patient will die within a few minutes. If someone is available with the training and proper equipment (highly unlikely), they could perform a formal endotracheal intubation (inserting a hollow breathing tube into the airway) or open the airway and insert a breathing tube via an incision in the neck (cricothyroidotomy) to save the patient. Either of these would have to be accomplished within 3–4 minutes after complete airway obstruction to avoid death or irreversible brain damage. Thankfully, however, such a scenario is an unusual occurrence in the wilderness setting.

If you can't clear the airway at first, keep trying. Breathing—either spontaneous (the patient's own efforts) or artificial (rescuer assisted)—is not possible without an open airway.

Once the patency (openness) of the airway is established, the rescuer should proceed with breathing assessment.

STEP 2: BREATHING

Few of us give much thought to the breathing process. But, in reality, breathing is complicated and at times counterintuitive. The first step is understanding a bit about the thoracic anatomy and how it functions. The lungs are housed in a strong but flexible cage—the rib cage—which is more or less cylindrical. Above the rib cage are the strong muscles of the neck, and below the rib cage are the broad diaphragm muscles. Between each rib are intercostal muscles.

The breathing cycle begins with contraction of the two diaphragm muscles (right and left), which expand the thoracic cylinder toward the abdomen and allow the lungs to expand. The muscles between the ribs (intercostal muscles) also contract to help lift the rib cage. This sequence represents inhalation (breathing in). Exhalation (breathing out) occurs when the diaphragm muscles relax and the strong intercostal muscles, which stretched during inhalation, spring back to their natural contracted state. Putting this all together, inhalation is an active process, while exhalation is generally considered a passive one. Although it is obviously possible to forcefully exhale, this is not part of a normal respiratory cycle.

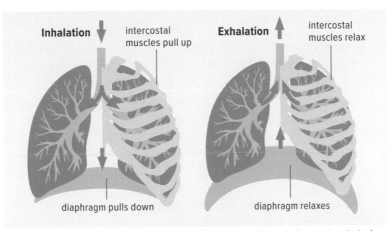

A simplified view of inhalation and exhalation.

Inhalation allows ambient air to enter the lungs for oxygen to be passed from the tiny air sacs (alveoli) in the lungs to the bloodstream, as well as to allow carbon dioxide to be discharged from the bloodstream into the alveoli, where it is expelled back into the atmosphere during exhalation. We have a tendency to view the acquisition of oxygen (inspiration) to be more important than ridding the body of carbon dioxide (expiration), but in reality, they are both equally important.

ASSESSING RESPIRATORY FUNCTION

After the airway has been assessed and cleared, the breathing assessment for a patient who is unconscious or in obvious distress is as follows:

1) Remove enough clothing so that both sides of the chest cavity are visible enough to accurately evaluate the respiratory cycle. Keep modesty and hypothermia concerns in mind as you do so.

2) **Look, Listen, Feel.** This will be repeated many times in this text, not only for breathing assessment, but also for the evaluation of almost all organ systems.

   Look at both sides of the chest during respiration. Do they move normally and symmetrically? How many times per minute is the patient breathing? Is the patient using muscles not normally used during respiration to breathe, such as the neck muscles? These are called accessory muscles of respiration, and they can be a very sensitive indicator that a person is experiencing severe respiratory distress and may even be at the point of imminent respiratory failure. When these muscles activate, it is a very dramatic presentation—the patient's neck muscles contract forcefully with each inspiration, and they can have a very panicked facial expression.

   Listen, either with the naked ear or with a stethoscope if you have one and know how to use it. If not, listen for abnormal sounds that may indicate respiratory distress. These would include wheezing (high-pitched sounds usually heard both on inhalation and exhalation), stridor (lower-pitched sounds from the trachea or larger airways), or other less-common sounds. You don't need to be a pulmonologist to accurately characterize the sounds—just use the adjectives that come to mind as you listen and then try to identify where in the chest they come from.

   Feel. Gently palpate (tap) the entire chest cavity to identify wounds, broken ribs, or any other indication of trauma.

Age Group	Age	Normal Respiratory Rate (Beats Per Minute)
1	1 year	30–40
2	2–5 years	20–40
3	6–10 years	15–25
4	11–18 years	15–20
5	18–70 years	12–20
6	>70 years	15–20

Even if you lack equipment or advanced training, there are a few maneuvers that will help to maximize a patient's pulmonary status until help arrives. First, place the patient in a position that makes it easiest to breathe. This will usually be with the head and torso elevated and aligned with each other, which allows the chest cavity to expand and contract with the least possible effort. Remember to be attentive to the possibility of the patient vomiting and aspirating (inhaling vomit into the lungs); to avoid this, place the patient slightly on one side.

If the breathing issue stems from a pre-existing medical issue, ask them or a companion if they normally use an inhaler or other medication. If they do, ask them if they should use it. Unless you have advanced training, it is not advisable to administer medications on your own.

STEP 3: CIRCULATION

As for all bodily systems, it is important to take a step back and understand the basics of the circulatory system before one can accurately assess irregularities in the system. If we don't understand these fundamentals, it becomes as easy to misdiagnose an insignificant problem as a serious one and vice versa.

Our circulatory system is nothing more than a closed, liquid-filled series of tubes driven by a cyclical pump. The tubes are veins and arteries, and the pump is the heart. Arteries conduct oxygenated, nutrient-rich blood from the heart to the various organs, and veins return the blood back to the heart, liver, and lungs. This returning blood has been stripped of oxygen and is transporting carbon dioxide and other toxins back to be filtered and expelled prior to being reoxygenated and recirculated. This cyclical pattern occurs as the heart pumps out blood, then pauses to refill.

UNDERSTANDING BLOOD PRESSURE AND HEART RATE

When a blood-pressure cuff is applied to the arm, it measures this cycle as two numbers: systolic blood pressure (the highest number, which reflects the forceful outflow of blood from the heart), and diastolic blood pressure (the refilling phase of the heart). A typical blood pressure reading would be 120/80. The typical units are represented in millimeters of mercury (mm/Hg). The average of these two is called the Mean Arterial Pressure, or MAP. For example, someone with a blood pressure of 120/80 would have a Mean Arterial Pressure of 100.

To put it another way, the alternating current in our homes functions in a very similar way. This cycle in our bodies repeats on average 60–80 times per minute. This number represents our pulse or heart rate.

Another important consideration is the amount of blood in the body. Although the actual quantity varies depending on the size of the individual, an average adult body has about five liters of blood (about 1.3 gallons). This concept will be explained further during the discussion regarding major trauma (see page 111).

There are several factors to consider when assessing the circulatory system. The most obvious aspect for trauma victims is identifying/recognizing internal and external bleeding and doing whatever is possible to slow or stop blood loss. Specific maneuvers to accomplish this will be reviewed again in the major trauma section of this text. The basic components of this initial circulatory examination consist of a rapid head-to-toe review with the Look, Listen, Feel structure mentioned on page 6. Areas of potential major blood loss include the neck, thorax, abdomen, pelvis, and the large arteries and veins of the extremities close to the torso.

After doing all we can to control bleeding, we transition to measuring and recording the patient's vital signs. For our purposes, vital signs include respiratory rate, pulse rate, and blood pressure. A concept that will be stressed in this text is the importance of not only measuring an initial set of vital signs, but also remeasuring them at frequent intervals, especially for a protracted extraction and/or a critically injured, unstable patient.

Age*	Resting Heart Rate (Beats Per Minute)	Blood Pressure
Newborn	100–150	65/40
Infant	100–150	95/60
Toddler	80–120	100/64
Child	75–115	110/60
Adolescent	60–100	120/80
Adult	60–100	120/80

*Keep in mind the above numbers represent averages. Numbers only slightly outside the above ranges shouldn't be cause for too much concern. Numbers that vary significantly should be reassessed for accuracy and treated appropriately.

CPR

Cardiopulmonary Resuscitation (CPR) represents the final attempt to save an individual whose heart and lungs have stopped functioning either from trauma or some medical catastrophe.

At this point, the patient's heart has stopped initiating an electric impulse, which, in turn, has caused the pumping chambers of the heart to cease the rhythmic distribution of blood around the body's circulatory system. This prevents the organs from receiving fresh, oxygenated blood, and the toxic metabolites of normal cellular function are no longer collected and taken away for disposal. This pump shutdown causes rapid unconsciousness and leads to death of the patient in just a few minutes if circulation of oxygenated blood cannot be reestablished within that time frame.

If we closely consider the catastrophic events that preceded the need for CPR and examine exactly what we hope to accomplish with chest compressions and artificial respirations, then the rationale is as follows:

CPR is an attempt to provide circulation (and oxygen) artificially. Unfortunately, unless the cardiac electrical system is rebooted, much the same way as a computer is rebooted, the compressions and rescue breathing often ultimately prove unsuccessful. This is why it is vitally important that an electric shocking device called an **Automatic Electric Defibrillator (AED)** becomes available within a few minutes of initiating CPR.

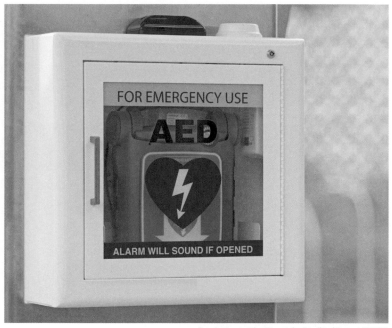

An Automatic Electric Defibrillator (AED)

Once it has been established that a patient has no pulse and is no longer breathing, CPR should begin immediately. Again, we should take the situation in context, meaning if you come across a pulseless, apneic (not breathing) patient without a witness to the event, it is a judgment call whether or not to initiate CPR. If the patient has obvious, nonsurvivable trauma; has obviously been dead for a long period of time; or manifests some other outward sign of nonviability, CPR may be withheld.

Another caveat to consider is that patients who suffer cardiopulmonary arrest due to trauma, especially blunt trauma, have a survival rate that approaches zero regardless of whether they are in a level 1 trauma center or in the backcountry. For this reason, unless there is a rescuer with advanced medical training present and definitive medical care is very close, CPR may also be withheld if a patient has suffered the arrest due to obvious massive trauma. One situation to be careful of is a patient who may appear to have suffered an arrest due to trauma but really experienced a medical event compounded by a subsequent trauma. A common example of this is a patient who suffers a cardiac arrest while driving and is found by rescuers to be in cardiopulmonary arrest and manifests signs of trauma as well. It can be extremely difficult in such a situation to determine the cause of the arrest. In this circumstance, it is advisable to initiate CPR unless obvious nonsurvivable trauma has been sustained by the patient.

CPR SPECIFICS

A convenient mnemonic device to use for patients suspected to have suffered a life-threatening medical event such as a myocardial infarction is **Check, Call, Care.** The details are explained below and summarized at the end of this chapter on page 20. If a patient appears to have suffered a recent cardiopulmonary arrest, the rescuers should assess the scene as they approach to ascertain that they are not placing themselves and other potential rescuers in a dangerous situation. Once this is established, any companions of the patient should be very quickly interrogated with only a few basic questions:

- What happened?
- How long have they been down?
- Do they have any underlying health conditions?
- Do they take any medications, and have any been skipped today?

These questions should be asked at the same time as the rescuer is assessing the victim. This should be done as follows: with the patient lying on a flat, hard surface in a supine position (on the back), the rescuer should kneel at the patient's side and feel for the inguinal (also called femoral; in the groin area) pulse while looking for any signs of spontaneous respirations. Chest rise and fall, or any lip or nasal movement, would indicate the patient is attempting to breathe on their own. If no pulse or respirations are noted within 10 seconds, the CPR sequence should be initiated.

A rescue call should be placed to 911, if possible, either by cell phone, satellite communication device, or by a runner if no other means are available. Again, the patient should be supine on a hard, flat surface. This is important to provide a backstop so that, during compressions, the chest cavity is efficiently compressed. The airway should be ascertained to be free of obstruction by quickly rolling the patient to one side and sweeping the mouth in a side-to-side fashion with a gloved finger. Strip any clothing away so that nothing is between the rescuer's hand and the patient's skin. Place the palm of one hand on the sternum directly between the nipples. This should be roughly 3–5 centimeters above (toward the patient's head) the connection of the ribs and the inferior (toward the patient's feet) aspect of the sternum.

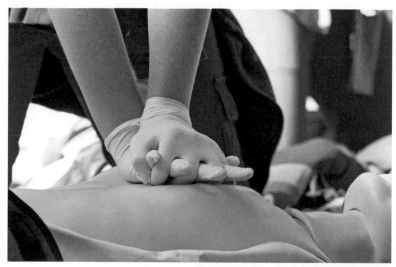

Proper hand position for performing CPR

Place the palm of the other hand directly on top of the hand that is on the patient's chest and interlock fingers. With elbows locked, begin compressions by bending at the waist and using your body weight to compress the patient's chest approximately 2–3 inches. This requires a tremendous amount of force to accomplish correctly. The ergonomic idea behind these mechanics is that the relatively small arm muscles are not the engine behind these rapid, repetitive, dynamic movements; rather, the large trunk muscles power the movements through the straight-line bones of the arms. Even the strongest bodybuilder would fatigue very rapidly if he did not utilize these precise body mechanics. The rate of compressions is the same for all ages from infants to the elderly: 100–120 compressions per minute. It is extremely helpful for someone not directly involved in the resuscitation process to call out the timing by using their cell phone or the timing function on their watch (100–120 beats per minute represents a compression every 0.5–0.7 seconds or so).

This level of exertion will tire a rescuer very quickly, so not only is it critical to use good body mechanics, but also that additional personnel are available to spell the person performing compressions. To this end, it would be a good idea to organize the available rescuers so that when the first individual becomes fatigued, the next person is already in position so that compressions are not interrupted for any length of time. (Two minutes is the recommended interval. Research has shown that the quality of CPR degrades quickly after this time period.) Again, it has been well documented that interruptions in chest compressions longer than 10 seconds corresponds to a marked decrease in survival.

Of equal importance is to allow complete recoil of the chest cavity between compressions. This allows the blood vessels on the surface of the heart that actually supply blood to the heart muscle to completely fill during each cycle. It is also helpful to have a spotter monitor these mechanics so that they can provide real-time feedback to the compressor.

Especially in the elderly population, broken ribs and a broken sternum are more common than not when CPR is performed correctly. This can be extraordinarily disconcerting for those with limited to no experience with resuscitations. In this setting, these broken bones are inconsequential and should be ignored.

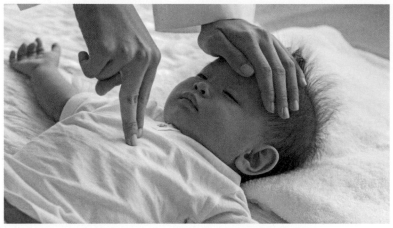

Performing chest compressions on an infant requires only one's fingers.

CPR ON PEDIATRIC PATIENTS

Pediatric patients should receive a proportionately diminished compressive force for their body size. Infants require compressions with only two to three fingers (see image above). The force applied should be graduated depending on chest depth. The palm of one hand, or a light touch with the standard two-hand technique would be appropriate for these patients. Again, the compressions should be just deep enough to propel blood from the heart so that it may be felt by a rescuer at the inguinal position.

CHECKING FOR A PULSE

If sufficient personnel are available, one person should kneel on the patient's side to feel for an inguinal pulse. This area is the most readily accessible and consistent place to locate a pulse. The exact location is just at the crease of the hip between the pubic bone and the laterally positioned hip bone (ASIS). Each compression should be forceful enough to pump blood from the heart to this inguinal pulse spot so that the pulse is easily felt. If no pulse is felt here, confirm with an additional rescuer, if possible, that the location is correct. If so, then the compressions are not of sufficient depth and the compressor should be instructed to compress deeper or should be replaced if fatigued.

People will often attempt to check for a pulse at the carotid artery in the neck. This location is notoriously difficult to detect due to the cross-hatched neck muscles that protect this vital structure. No such overlying tissue exists in the inguinal region.

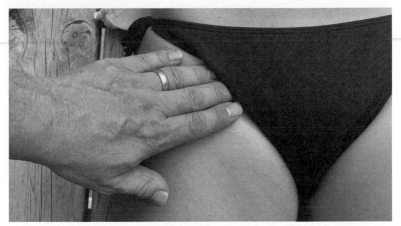

Modesty is of secondary importance in this setting.

After 30 compressions are delivered, rescue breathing should be instituted as follows:

An additional rescuer should deliver two deep breaths via a mouth-to-mouth technique in adults. This should be accomplished while simultaneously pinching the nose shut so that the newly delivered breath does not simply exit out of the patient's nose. In infants and toddlers, the rescuer's mouth should be placed completely over the mouth and nose so that the delivered air is forced into both the victim's mouth as well as the nares.

A WORD ABOUT RESCUE BREATHING

Delivering rescue breaths in a direct mouth-to-mouth fashion is certainly uncomfortable for a rescuer to perform on a stranger and may also place the rescuer at some risk for acquiring a transmissible disease. Two options exist to mitigate this problem. The first is to avoid rescue breaths altogether, the so-called "compression only" technique for CPR. If the rescuer(s) feels uncomfortable with direct mouth-to-mouth contact, this represents an acceptable (albeit somewhat less effective) technique. The second option is to utilize some sort of barrier device. There are multiple options on the market, but they all function to prevent direct skin contact. An

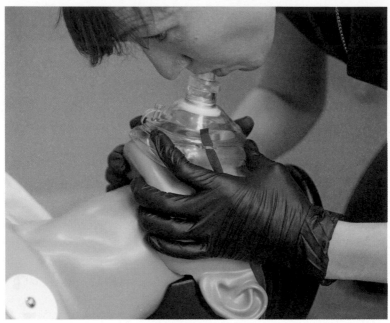
Rescue breaths being delivered to a CPR dummy using a barrier device

example of a barrier device that can be clipped to a keychain or backpack is shown above. It would be highly unusual for such a device to be available in a timely fashion unless a rescuer happened to carry one in a first aid kit. It should be emphasized that chest compressions are the most important component of CPR, so the rescuers should not feel pressured

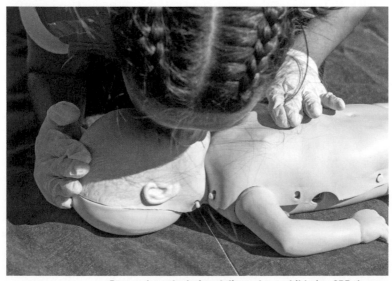
Rescue breaths being delivered to a child-size CPR dummy

to provide direct mouth-to-mouth breaths if they do not feel comfortable doing so.

This cycle of 30:2 should be continued. The team should also check that the patient's chest rises significantly with each rescue breath. If not, tilt the head back slightly and retry.

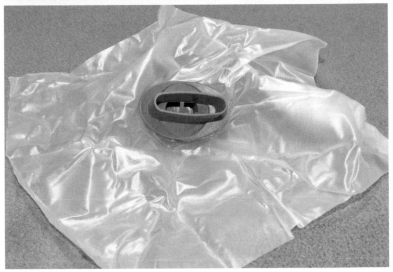

A rescue breathing barrier with a one-way valve

AUTOMATED EXTERNAL DEFIBRILLATORS (AEDS) AND HOW TO USE THEM

Additionally, communication should be ongoing with requests for more trained personnel, oxygen, and, most importantly, an AED. It is impossible to overstate how time-sensitive this treatment algorithm is. Every minute that passes allows for more cardiac muscle to become ischemic (deprived of oxygenated blood). This in turn will lead to the death of the affected muscle and a diminished probability of recovery. The administration of supplemental oxygen either via nasal cannula, face mask, or through an endotracheal tube inserted by trained personnel through the mouth and vocal cords will help improve this ischemic process.

The AED represents a vital component in this process. This device consists of a small computer that senses electrical activity by way of two gel pads that are affixed to the patient's bare skin. These pads sense cardiac electrical activity and relay this information to the computer. If the

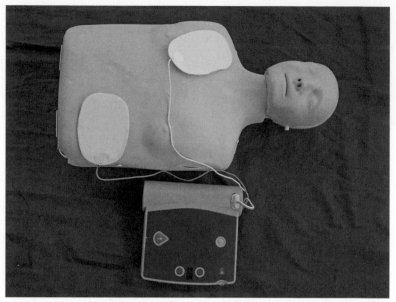

An AED showing the correct positioning of the electrical pads.

computer detects an appropriate electric environment, it delivers a brief but powerful electric pulse through these same cables and pads. The concept is that this sudden electric pulse will reawaken the patient's own cardiac conduction system and that the heart will start to initiate its own normal electric impulses.

When the AED unit arrives at the patient, place it close to the patient's head and turn it on first, as it can take several minutes to initialize. Next, remove the pads from the case. These should be attached to cables that are, in turn, attached to the main unit. The first pad should be placed on the patient's chest just below the right collarbone, while the second is positioned low on the left lateral (side) aspect of the chest. Take care to ensure that this pad is not placed too low. It should be situated directly over the rib cage. Again, the skin must be dry before pad placement. Turn on the device. There should be a laminated summary tag attached to the machine. This should be quickly read beforehand if the rescuer is not familiar with the device. Some machines will automatically sense the cardiac rhythm and deliver a shock if appropriate. Others require a switch to be activated before this occurs. If nothing happens, confer with a partner to ensure that it is being used properly. It is important that

CPR stops and that no one touches either the patient or anything that is touching the patient so that a collateral shock is not inadvertently delivered to rescue personnel.

Whether or not a shock is delivered, leave the pads attached and continue CPR if no inguinal pulse is felt and/or the patient does not begin to breathe spontaneously. Most machines will automatically reassess for a shockable rhythm at 2-minute intervals. If this does not seem to be occurring, have someone set a recurring timer on a smartphone or watch and manually reset the machine every 2 minutes.

AED Use for Pediatric Patients

Most AED packages will come with pediatric gel pads and have pediatric settings on the device. Children require less energy to deliver an effective defibrillating pulse. For this application, the age/weight cutoff is typically 8 years and 55 pounds. If pediatric pads and/or settings are not available, use the adult pads and, if possible, manually adjust the AED to deliver the minimal possible energy (joules).

WHEN TO STOP CPR

Although peer-reviewed data are somewhat sparse for the topic of survival statistics for backcountry CPR, the consensus is that less than 10% of patients who suffer cardiopulmonary arrest outside of an urban setting survive even with timely, appropriate resuscitative attempts. This percentage represents a compendium of all patients who suffer cardiopulmonary arrest in the field. There are subgroups, such as hypothermic drowning and indirect lightning strike victims, who survive at a much higher rate. Therefore, CPR should be initiated as rapidly as possible and continued while attempts to obtain a pertinent history are underway.

There is no exact time frame to dictate when to stop CPR. Without signs of life, unless the patient has been extremely hypothermic, the survival rate beyond 30 minutes of continuous resuscitative efforts is essentially zero. At this point, a final check for spontaneous pulse and respirations should be done, the AED should be tried one last time, and, if this is unsuccessful, the patient may be declared dead.

Obviously, all situations present their own unique challenges and circumstances that may well direct either a longer or shorter course of CPR. Rescuer exhaustion, rescuer safety, an obviously nonviable patient, and other considerations may prompt the rescue personnel to stop the rescue efforts after only a few minutes. Conversely, bystander history of a witnessed arrest, child with a submersion event, impending arrival of personnel with advanced training and equipment, or other findings may call for a longer trial of CPR.

SUMMARY

Check If you encounter a patient who has apparently suffered a medical or traumatic event that has resulted in cardiopulmonary arrest, quickly assess the area for rescuer safety and to ascertain the circumstances surrounding the event. Ask the victim's companions, if available. After scene safety is ensured, check for an inguinal pulse for 10 seconds while inspecting the airway/chest cavity for spontaneous respirations.

Call If no pulse or respirations are detected, call 911 or otherwise send for assistance.

Care After quickly turning the patient on their side and clearing the airway, roll the patient back to supine and start chest compressions as described above at a rate of 100/minute. After 30 compressions, deliver 2 rescue breaths while continuing chest compressions with the head of the patient tilted back slightly (so-called sniffing position) while an additional rescuer checks for an inguinal pulse. If none is detected, continue the 30:2 cycle until the patient revives, advanced trained personnel arrive, the patient is declared deceased, or factors such as exhaustion prompt the rescuer(s) to stop.

FIELD REPORT

A 49-year-old male slumps unconscious while being top-roped on an ice climb. He quickly falls to an upside-down position and is hanging from his climbing harness. This event is witnessed by multiple personnel, including several WFR-trained individuals and a neurosurgeon who is climbing nearby. Several climbing guides who are working in the same area quickly rig a separate rope system and haul the stricken climber about 20 feet to the top of the cliff and away from the cliff's edge. By this time, EMS personnel are hiking in with ACLS (Advanced Cardio-pulmonary Life Support) knowledge and equipment. After detecting no signs of life, the neurosurgeon directs that CPR be initiated. CPR continues for approximately 10 minutes until EMS personnel arrive. The patient is intubated and ventilated by hand-bagging with 100% oxygen while cardiac compressions continue. Multiple rounds of ACLS medications are administered intravenously and signs of life are looked for at 5-minute intervals. An AED is appropriately affixed to the patient's bare, dry skin, but no shockable rhythm is detected. EMS personnel confirm that the unit is working properly. The device continues to reset and check for a shockable rhythm every 2 minutes. No such rhythm is detected. Additional personnel with advanced training arrives at about the 40-minute mark. At 50 minutes, CPR is halted along with artificial ventilation. The AED is activated one last time and a final round of cardiac drugs is administered. No signs of life are detected and, after agreement with the two doctors present, the patient is pronounced deceased.

Takeaways

- Patient is immediately transferred to a hard, flat surface in an area that is safe for rescuers.

- 911 is called in this circumstance even before assessment has begun. It is obvious that the patient will require highly trained personnel, and, due to the remote location, an early call will avoid a long delay before their arrival.

- CPR is started immediately.

- Due to the patient's young age, the witnessed arrest, and the fact that a component of hypothermia may be present, CPR is continued for 50 minutes.

CHOKING AND THE HEIMLICH MANEUVER

Earlier in this chapter, we detailed the importance of clearing the airway for traumatic and medical conditions, but in this section, we will specifically cover what to do when someone is choking. If we inadvertently inhale food or other objects into the trachea instead of swallowing them down the esophagus and into the stomach, we are at risk for that object lodging at the level of the vocal cords which, in turn, causes us to choke.

Such objects may cause a complete or partial obstruction of the airway. Either way, the situation is an emergency, but complete, untreated airway blockage will result in death in only a few minutes. Rapid recognition and intervention become vital in order to save the person's life.

Signs and Symptoms of Partial Airway Obstruction

- Violent coughing

- Extreme difficulty with both inhalation and exhalation

- Hoarseness or inability to speak

Signs and Symptoms of Complete Airway Obstruction

- Inability to exchange air either in or out

- Inability to make any sound

- Extreme panic

- Clutching throat with hands

TREATMENT

If the patient is coughing and able to exchange sufficient air, give them space and allow them to attempt to cough it out. If this is not successful within a minute or so, emergency personnel should be called if available. If in the backcountry, continue to allow them to try to expel the object on their own unless their clinical condition deteriorates or they lose consciousness. At this point, intervention as per complete obstruction should be implemented.

For complete obstruction, treatment should begin immediately. If the victim is conscious and upright, stand behind

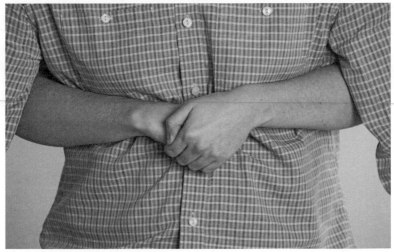

Figure 1

the patient and lock hands by forming a fist with one hand and then wrapping it with the other. Place the thumb side of the fist hand directly below the bottom of the breastbone (sternum). An extremely forceful, violent thrusting of the joined hands should be performed. This will require essentially all the strength of most rescuers. Ideally, the thrust should be timed with the patient's attempt at exhalation. Continue this process until the object is ejected out of the airway (see Figure 1 above). If the patient is unconscious, ensure that no residual foreign objects remain by placing the patient on his or her side while lying down and sweeping the mouth with a gloved finger (if possible) in a side-to-side motion.

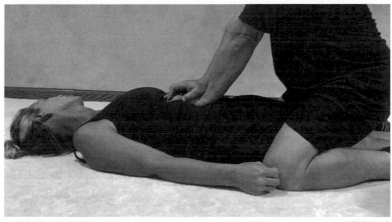

Figure 2

If the patient is unconscious, otherwise on the ground, or much larger than the rescuer, the patient should lie on their back while the rescuer straddles the patient and delivers sharp upward thrusts with the palms. The fingers will be intertwined as per the hand position for performing CPR. However, instead of placing the hands on top of the sternum, the rescuer should position their linked hands below the breastbone and aim forceful thrusts more toward the victim's head (see Figure 2 on page 23).

Infants and Children

Children older than 3 or so are treated the same way as choking adults. Obviously, proportionally less force must be used to avoid injury (see Figure 3).

Toddlers and infants are treated a bit differently in that they are easy to pick up. This allows gravity to help us expel the lodged object. The child may be picked up by the feet or placed on the forearm with mouth toward the ground. Several sharp blows between the shoulder blades are administered. This should be continued again until the object is dislodged (see Figure 4).

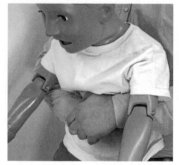
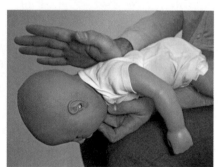

Figure 3 Figure 4

This section will cover medical topics that, while not necessarily life-threatening, will still require field management. There is an almost infinite number of minor medical issues that may crop up in the outdoors. We will cover some of the more common ones. Hopefully, if you encounter a situation that is not covered here, you can figure out what to do based on the information provided.

RASHES AND SKIN CONDITIONS

Many plants in North America and around the world produce irritating and/or toxic substances on their surfaces to deter herbivores from eating them. Unfortunately for us, these substances may produce skin reactions that can be quite painful—even debilitating in some cases. Recognition and avoidance are the most effective means of preventing these rashes (called contact dermatitis), but pants, long sleeves, and even gloves will help prevent exposure if one must pass through an environment rich in toxic plants. Some of the more common plants are listed below.

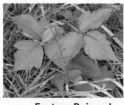
Eastern Poison Ivy

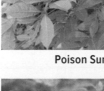
Poison Sumac

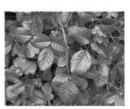
Poison Oak

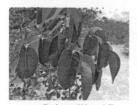
Poison Wood Tree

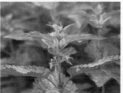
Stinging Nettle

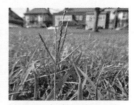
Many varieties of grasses, such as Bermuda Grass

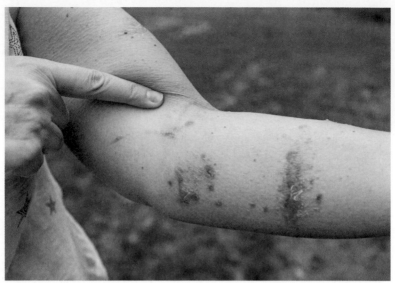
A rash after exposure to Poison Ivy

The list may extend to up to several hundred types of plants that may cause contact dermatitis in susceptible individuals. The best policy is to avoid skin contact or ingestion of any plant unless you're absolutely sure that it is safe.

Most individuals exposed to poison ivy, poison sumac, or poison oak develop a florid allergic reaction where the leaf of the plant contacts the skin. This reaction is called a delayed hypersensitivity reaction and typically appears within minutes to hours of exposure. The toxin is an oil-based chemical, so washing with soap as soon as possible is essential to limit the damage. The soap will emulsify the oily toxin so that the water may wash it away.

The reaction can vary from mild to extremely severe. Highly susceptible individuals may develop a raised, dripping wound that lasts for several weeks.

Besides immediate washing of the area with soap, the affected individual should remove any clothing that may have potentially come into contact with the plant and wash them with soap and warm water. Care must be taken to avoid touching the eyes or mucous membranes if any hint of residual oil is on the fingers.

All plants that cause allergic dermatitis may produce severe reactions, but the oil-based toxins usually produce the more serious injuries.

Treatment of the condition involves washing as mentioned above, wrapping the area loosely with a breathable gauze, taking ibuprofen, and seeking medical care for more serious/extensive exposures. Topical creams or ointments are generally not helpful for these types of reactions, but you can try a topical over-the-counter hydrocortisone cream for short periods of time (up to 2–3 days). Some people have found calamine lotion or similar products useful to minimize the discomfort and itching.

SUNBURN

The term *sunburn* is really just a colloquialism for a first-degree burn. This phenomenon is almost always a result of prolonged exposure of unprotected skin to the sun's rays. These effects are pronounced at high altitudes where the atmosphere is thinner and thus offers less protection from the damaging UV (ultraviolet) rays, as well as closer to the equator where people tend to spend longer periods outdoors with large surface areas of uncovered skin.

Obviously, the best form of treatment is prevention. Sunscreen provides adequate protection under most circumstances, as long as it is reapplied frequently. Sweating and water submersion will wash away sunscreen, so even more frequent reapplication must be performed.

A more effective prevention method is covering all exposed skin with clothing or other barriers so that there is no way for the UV rays to directly contact the skin. High-altitude mountaineers must be especially conscious of this potentially serious problem. Negligent exposure to the intense solar rays at altitude may result in burns that go beyond the typical epidermal searing to include damage to deeper tissues. Another issue to be considered when traveling on snow, glaciers, or water is that the solar rays reflected off these surfaces will travel upward and may render the protection of wide-brimmed hats and other single-layered garments useless.

It should be noted that even darker-skinned individuals are at risk for sunburn.

The treatment for sunburn consists mostly of supportive care and preventing re-exposure. Adequate oral hydration is essential, especially for larger burns that encompass more

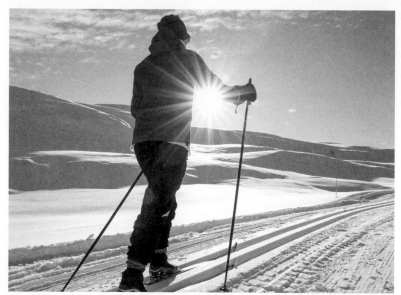
Sunburn isn't just a concern at the beach; at high elevations it's a serious concern as well.

of the body's surface area. Commercially available after-sun creams that contain aloe may help relieve some of the pain, but the skin will take at least several days to heal by shedding damaged outer layers and replacing them with new, fresh ones.

BRUISES AND SCRAPES

Minor damage to the skin and underlying tissues occurs with minimal force traumas such as falls from standing or other relatively low-energy-transferring events.

Scrapes are superficial breaches in the skin as a result of such events. Treatment includes covering them with nonstick bandages and allowing the damaged tissue to slough and be replaced by regenerated cells from beneath in a similar fashion as the healing process for sunburns. Topical ointments and oral antibiotics are not needed for these minor injuries.

A **bruise** represents a hemorrhage beneath the skin as a result of a mild blunt-force event. The overlying skin usually remains intact. Again, healing will occur using the body's regenerative capacities. The blood will be reabsorbed in days to weeks and be recycled. Ice, elevation, and ibuprofen will help with the discomfort and swelling.

BLISTERS

Blisters represent yet another spectacular way in which the body tries to protect itself from environmental insults. When a spot on the skin surface is irritated by, say, the constant back-and-forth motion of the inside of an ill-fitting shoe on the heel, the body will send pain signals to the brain as a warning for the individual to stop and address the problem. If this warning is not heeded, the body takes matters into its own hands by sacrificing the superficial layers of skin. It does this by causing clear fluid (interstitial fluid) to accumulate between this superficial skin layer and the deeper, more important tissues. The result is a blister. This blister acts in much the same way as an airbag in a car. The airbag deploys to protect the occupant.

There are limits, however, to the effectiveness of this protective mechanism. Continued neglect of the causative condition will break the blister and lead to damage of the sub-epidermal tissues.

When a blister is recognized, it is best to stop and fix the underlying issue. This may include tightening shoes or adding or subtracting a layer of sock. Additionally, the blister should be left intact, if possible, and covered with a bandage. If the blister is too large and the foot cannot be placed comfortably back in the shoe, the fluid may be drained with a sterilized needle prior to placing the dressing. It is advisable to leave the overlying skin intact, if possible, to provide an additional layer of protection.

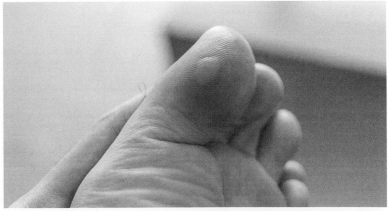

A blister, a common backcountry ailment

CRAMPS

While there exists no medical consensus as to the actual cause of muscle cramping, many theories exist to explain this painful and transient phenomenon. The prevailing reasoning is that a lack of potassium during exercise causes muscles to cramp and seize up. The fact is that the body does a remarkable job of maintaining electrolyte equilibrium even during intense exercise; however, as with all compensatory bodily regulatory mechanisms, there are limits to these auto-adjustments.

A more likely explanation is that a combination of factors, such as depletion of intracellular energy sources, dehydration, and perhaps some electrolyte depletion and/or excess, causes the issue. Whatever the cause, the treatment is fairly simple: stop the exercise and engage in gentle stretching, rehydration, and rest. The addition of a reasonable quantity of electrolyte solution containing potassium, sodium, and magnesium can also help.

DEHYDRATION

Anyone who has worked hard outdoors in the garden or in the backcountry on a hot day has probably experienced at least a

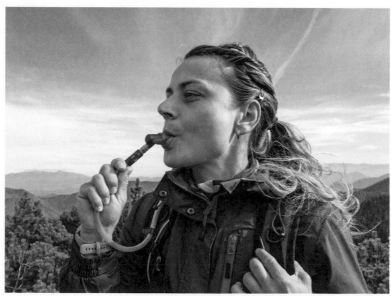

Adequate hydration is essential but easy to overlook.

mild case of dehydration. Our bodies do a marvelous job of maintaining what is called fluid and electrolyte homeostasis. What this means is that if we exert ourselves and lose fluids either through sweat or through an increased rate of respiration, our internal sensors send signals to cells to release additional fluid into the bloodstream to compensate. The same is true for electrolytes such as sodium and potassium. These losses must be replenished quickly, however, or we face becoming dehydrated.

Except for extreme cases of dehydration, these losses are easily replaced by pausing the exertion and drinking a combination of water and water with electrolyte additives. It requires some time for the body to assimilate and redistribute the fluids and electrolytes, so patience is needed to regain a healthy internal environment. The progression of signs and symptoms of dehydration are listed below:

Mild

- Increased thirst
- Excessive sweating

Moderate to Severe

- Extreme thirst
- Diminished/absent sweating
- Light-headedness
- Weakness
- Delirium
- Coma/Death

As with all preventable conditions, adequate preparation and early recognition and treatment are essential.

MILD SPRAINS

Although the term sprain is used frequently in the lay medical lexicon to allude to a rather vague set of conditions, the word has a specific meaning. All joints in the body are held together by surrounding ligaments and tendons, the

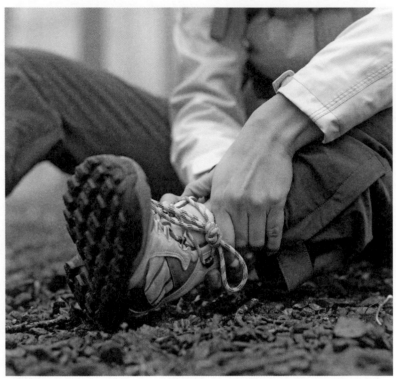
Sprains are among the most common injuries.

difference being that ligaments attach two or more bones together while tendons attach muscle to bone. Both are integral to maintain joint stability.

When a body part such as a knee or foot is moved violently in a direction counter to its design, then the supporting ligaments and/or tendons may suffer damage. The damage usually consists of a combination of severe stretching and partial tears of the affected structure. The underlying bones remain intact. The pain from such an injury may be severe. Other signs and symptoms include swelling, instability of the joint, and subcutaneous hemorrhage (bruising) that manifests as purplish discoloration around the affected joint.

Treatment includes taking measures to not reinjure the joint. For instance, walking on a sprained ankle is not recommended. Circumstances in the backcountry may require a person to walk on an injured part. In this case, splint the joint with whatever is available to limit ANY motion of the joint. One method is to use tape on both sides of an ankle or knee and then cover it with an elastic wrap.

The usual recommendation is **RICE—Rest, Ice, Compression** (loose to allow for additional swelling), and **Elevation**. It cannot be overstated how important it is to not overtighten a circumferential bandage and to reassess the adequacy of blood flow to the extremity distal to the compressive dressing. Again, checking capillary refill and pulses accomplish this requirement.

Sprains essentially never require any sort of operation or invasive intervention. They will heal over time, although in severe cases this may take weeks to months.

DENTAL EMERGENCIES

Dental emergencies, while typically not life-threatening, result in significant pain and a prematurely shortened backcountry experience. Listed below are some common dental issues that may be encountered within or outside city limits.

- Broken tooth
- Dental abscess
- Loss of filling or crown

Broken teeth, either from falls, direct facial blows, or biting a hard object, will certainly cause significant pain. This pain will be exacerbated by inhaling cold air or chewing on the affected area.

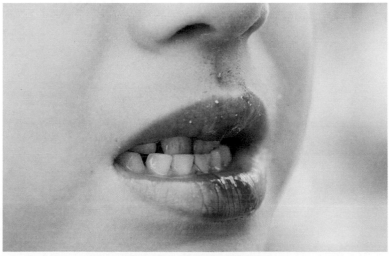

Dental injuries are relatively common, especially with children.

A very useful first aid item in the backcountry is a dental cream that may be used as a temporary covering over the injured tooth. These creams are typically available over the counter. A dollop of cream is placed on the fingertip and then liberally spread over the broken tooth. The cream will need to be reapplied after eating.

Dental abscesses occur when a caries (cavity) erodes into the supporting bone (maxilla or mandible) or the nerve beneath the tooth. These small pockets of purulence can be excruciating. The only effective field treatment consists of the administration of oral antibiotics and painkillers. A combination of acetaminophen and ibuprofen works very well for this condition. Antibiotics may be started if access to definitive dental care will be delayed more than 48 hours or so. Penicillin or amoxicillin work well for those without a penicillin allergy. Clindamycin works well for those unable to tolerate penicillin or its derivatives.

Loss of a filling or crown may also be treated with a dental filling cream. As for broken teeth, softs foods should be selected, and the food should stay in the unaffected side of the mouth.

Another trick, if dental cream is not available, to secure a dislodged crown is to use toothpaste. Apply a small dab to the crown, then compress the crown onto its origin tooth. This method will not be as secure as dental cream, so avoid chewing until definitive dental care is available.

MAJOR MEDICAL ISSUES

This chapter deals with the backcountry management of nontraumatic medical conditions, which are presented in descending order of severity and/or frequency. It should be noted that any medical condition that may affect an individual in urban areas may also do so in rural settings. On top of these possibilities exist many other conditions unique to the backcountry setting. Additionally, many illnesses that may not present significant diagnostic or treatment challenges in metropolitan areas may quickly become life-threatening when treatment and evacuation resources are limited.

The most important consideration in the management of medical calamities in a wilderness setting is to try to make the most accurate diagnosis possible. Doing so will provide the foundation for expeditious field treatment and evacuation planning.

Even for trained personnel, making an exact diagnosis of a medical condition may be difficult or even impossible without the appropriate technologies available in a hospital setting, but we will cover simple diagnostic algorithms that will hopefully allow a rescuer to make as accurate an assessment of the patient's condition as possible given backcountry resource limitations.

As discussed in the first chapter concerning the ABCs, any individual who appears to be suffering from a condition that could be potentially life-threatening must first receive a rapid ABC assessment. Further diagnostic maneuvers may be undertaken once these basics are covered.

HEART ATTACKS

As the pump that distributes oxygenated blood and retrieves toxic byproducts from every tissue in the body, the heart obviously represents a critical piece of machinery. When this pump fails to operate smoothly, even for brief periods, all bodily systems suffer. When catastrophic pump failure occurs, death ensues within a few minutes.

When we think of life-threatening cardiac conditions, we typically think first of heart attacks, or **myocardial infarctions (MIs)** as they are known in medical terms. Indeed, myocardial infarctions far and away represent the most common severe cardiac event that occurs in the backcountry. We will briefly explore cardiac anatomy and the alterations thereof.

Every single cell in the human body requires a continuous supply of oxygenated blood to function properly. Any failure of this delivery system, even for a few seconds, will cause a critical cascade of failure in the tissues that do not receive blood flow. In the case of the heart, when blood flow is interrupted in the arteries (which supply the heart muscle), the affected muscle begins to die. This is called a heart attack or myocardial infarction.

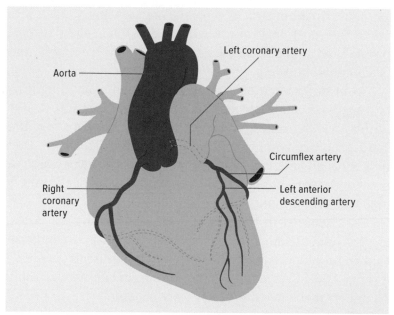

The arteries of the heart

When a blockage occurs in the small arteries, as shown above, the muscle beyond the blockage begins to die and a myocardial infarction has begun. The blockages are typically caused by a long-standing disruption in the lining of the artery that narrows the inside diameter of the artery. Additional factors such as dehydration, exertion, or cold exposure then lead to a favorable environment within the artery for the formation of blood clots. This typically represents the final step in the blockage of the vessel.

Symptoms of a Myocardial Infarction (MI)

- Severe chest pressure and/or pain. A classic description is an elephant sitting on the patient's chest.
- Pain radiating down the left arm and/or up into the left jaw
- Less commonly, pain radiating down the right arm and/or up into the right jaw
- Shortness of breath not explained by increased exertion or other causes
- Sweating also unaffiliated with increased exertion
- Sudden loss of consciousness with lack of spontaneous pulse and/or respirations. This is called a *sudden death* event. While other conditions may cause this (stroke, for example), myocardial infarctions represent far and away the most frequent cause.

Note that many atypical symptoms also occur. These symptoms may be very subtle and may even escape the attention of trained medical personnel. They include:

- Indigestion—in other words, a patient may feel a fullness or even acid reflux that is not associated with recent overeating.
- Nausea
- Pain in atypical locations, such as the back or upper stomach region

A FEW ADDITIONAL KEY POINTS TO KEEP IN MIND

We typically think of myocardial infarctions occurring in overweight, middle-aged to old men who exert themselves excessively. While this is indeed true, it is imperative to understand that essentially anyone may suffer a heart attack. Patients who suffer an acute cardiac event are frequently misdiagnosed even in hospital settings by physicians who disregard a patient's symptoms because they don't fit within the parameters of the classic patient profile.

Categories of patients who suffer from myocardial infarctions and who are frequently misdiagnosed include:

- Women

- Apparently fit individuals

- Young adults

In addition, risk factors that increase the odds that a patient will suffer a heart attack include:

- **Smoking**   This is far and away the number one risk factor that increases the incidence of blockage of the coronary arteries.

- **Obesity**   Obese individuals suffer fatal cardiac complications at a significantly increased rate as compared to lean individuals.

- **Family history**   Even lean, fit individuals who don't smoke may suffer a heart attack with more frequency than the general population due to genetic factors. There are even classes of individuals who routinely die from heart attacks in their 20s or 30s due to certain genetic conditions. It is therefore extremely important for a rescuer to obtain a brief, focused assessment of the patient's family history if they exhibit any of the signs or symptoms of a myocardial infarction. A simple direct question, such as "Have YOU or anyone in your family ever had a heart attack?" should suffice. Notice that the question includes asking the patient if they have ever experienced a heart attack.

FIELD ASSESSMENT AND TREATMENT

An individual who displays any of the signs or symptoms must be considered to be experiencing a heart attack until proven otherwise. Given the rapidity with which a blocked coronary artery causes irreversible cardiac muscle damage, treatment must be initiated immediately, even before a definitive diagnosis is made.

Field assessment consists of identifying the signs and symptoms, determining if they are compatible with a cardiac event, and initiating care. This should be done within a matter of seconds. Again, the mnemonic is **Check, Call (911), Care.**

Ideally, several rescuers will be available so that one individual does not have to perform all tasks. If the patient is experiencing a sudden death event as described above, CPR should be initiated immediately. Someone should transmit that information to authorities ASAP so that personnel with advanced training (ACLS—Advanced Cardiac Life Support) can be dispatched to the scene.

If patients are conscious, and with spontaneous respirations and pulse, they should be placed in a comfortable seated position that favors positive respiratory mechanics. They may be placed partially on their side if they are nauseated so that if they vomit, they don't aspirate the vomit into their lungs. If they routinely take any cardiac medications such as nitroglycerin, that may be administered as the patient or licensed provider instructs. A baby aspirin (81 mg—chewable 2–4 tablets) should be given to the patient, if available and no contraindications such as an allergy to aspirin exists. If the full 325 mg adult dose is all that is available, the patient should chew and swallow one of these. Oxygen should be acquired as soon as possible and administered either with a mask or by nose (nasal cannula). Any restrictive clothing should be loosened or removed. Immediate transport to an appropriate medical facility must be arranged on an urgent basis.

FIELD REPORT

A very fit 60-year-old male is mountain biking with his two sons in the mountains of southwest Colorado. He is a paramedic, an instructor for a rescue rigging company, and a long-term officer of the local search and rescue team. Midway into the ride, he complains of sudden chest pressure and difficulty breathing. As he and his sons discuss returning to the trailhead, he suddenly collapses and becomes unresponsive. His sons immediately call 911 and begin CPR. The rescue team arrives within 30 minutes and resuscitative efforts are continued for almost an hour without return of signs of life. He is pronounced dead at the scene.

There are several lessons to be learned here. First of all, fatal cardiac events can strike even the most seemingly healthy individuals. Therefore, a very high index of suspicion must be maintained in the presence of ANY symptoms compatible with a heart attack. It is much better to be proven wrong than to ignore a potentially life-ending event.

Secondly, CPR and then advanced lifesaving protocols must be initiated immediately. Although the aid rendered in this case did not improve the outcome, everything that could have been done was performed perfectly.

Lastly, and unfortunately, the vast majority of cardiac sudden death events are not survivable, but every endeavor to initiate CPR/AED assistance should be undertaken.

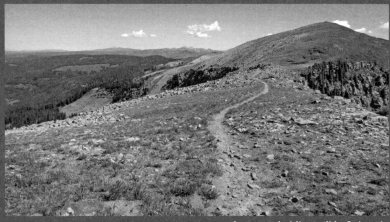

A mountain bike trail in Colorado

STROKES (CEREBROVASCULAR ACCIDENTS)

The term *stroke* is frequently used in the lay press to describe a certain condition that affects the brain, although stroke refers to a rather broad array of sudden-onset events that occur to the brain. The result of any of these events is that a section of the brain is suddenly deprived of its blood supply. When this occurs, the involved brain matter may suffer irreversible damage within only a few minutes. The physical manifestation of such damage depends entirely on which part of the brain is involved. The brain controls all bodily functions—both voluntary and involuntary. This means that the signs and symptoms of a stroke are numerous and may include a wide variety of physical alterations from very subtle all the way to death.

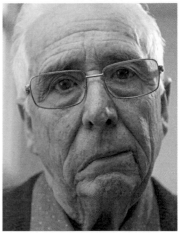
Weakness on one side of the body, including the face, is a sign of stroke.

Some of the More Common Signs and Symptoms of Stroke

- Weakness or complete loss of motor function on one side of the body (hemiparesis or hemiparalysis)

- Weakness of the muscles on one side of the face (facial droop)

- Confusion

- Difficulty speaking, or markedly altered speech (various types of aphasias)

- Vision changes—even blindness in one or both eyes

- Extreme headache

It bears repeating that some symptoms may be extremely subtle, so a high index of suspicion must be maintained. It can be very helpful to question a companion of the patient to see if the friend has noticed any changes.

The CDC has recommended a mnemonic for the rapid identification of a stroke in evolution. It is **FAST.**

F—Face   Ask the person to smile. If the corners of the mouth do not move symmetrically, a stroke is likely occurring.

A—Arms   Ask the person to raise both arms. If they cannot raise one arm, or an arm involuntarily drifts downward, a stroke is likely occurring.

S—Speech   Ask the person to repeat a simple phrase. If there is any difficulty with this, a stroke is likely occurring.

T—Time   If any one or more of the above is happening, the patient must be evacuated immediately to a facility that can manage an evolving stroke. This means the nearest medium-to-large hospital.

The reason for the extreme urgency is that some of the damage from a stroke may be limited or even reversed with expeditious treatment. There are medications and operative interventions that can be lifesaving if administered within a short time frame. For strokes, the golden hour is just that: within 60 minutes. Benefit may still be achieved after an hour, but the results dwindle rapidly as time goes on.

It is worthwhile to present a bit of anatomy and physiology information here so that rescuers may better understand what happens during a stroke event and may visualize what is occurring inside a patient's brain—and thus more fully understand the need for rapid evacuation and treatment.

The medical term for a stroke is a cerebrovascular accident (CVA). This correctly implies that the underlying problem is with the blood vessels that supply the brain with fresh, oxygenated blood. Three basic conditions cause this potentially devastating injury.

Hemorrhagic CVA   This condition occurs when a blood vessel bursts inside the skull, which in turn causes direct damage to the brain matter due to the pressure from the ruptured artery. These types of CVAs tend to produce devastating injuries and even death when they first occur.

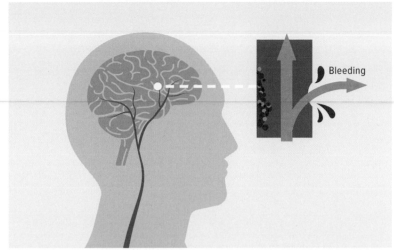

A hemorrhagic stroke occurs when blood leaks into the brain.

Thrombotic CVA These strokes are due to blood clots forming within the blood vessels in the brain. This situation is exactly the same as a clog in household plumbing—no water can flow past the obstruction. In the case of a thrombotic CVA, no blood can bypass the blockage, and all the brain tissue beyond (distal to) the obstruction is deprived of oxygenated blood and thus begins to die almost immediately. The severity of this variety of CVA is entirely dependent on how big and where the involved blood vessel is located.

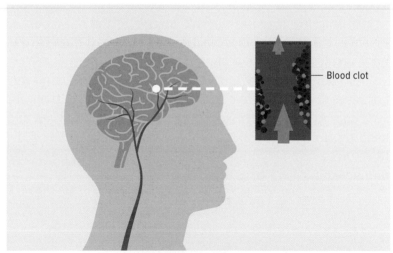

A thrombotic stroke occurs when a blood clot occurs in one of the blood vessels in the brain.

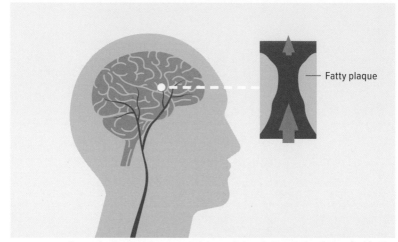

An embolic stroke occurs when a clot or fatty plaque is carried in the bloodstream from other areas in the body and then lodges in the smaller arteries of the brain.

Embolic CVA These events produce exactly the same sort of injury as thrombotic CVAs. The difference here is that instead of a primary clot that forms within the vessel, the obstruction is caused by a piece of solid material (such as a blood clot) that comes from somewhere else in the bloodstream and then becomes lodged in a cerebral vessel, which in turn occludes (obstructs) it. These sorts of strokes tend to be milder at initial presentation and often favor the vessels of the eyes. Affected patients frequently complain of visual changes or vision loss in one eye.

In practice, it really doesn't matter to the backcountry rescuer which of the above is the culprit, but it does help to have an idea of what is occurring in real time.

As mentioned above, rapid identification and air evacuation represent the two most important interventions for a rescuer to perform. In addition, supplemental oxygen and keeping the patient's head elevated above the level of the heart are extremely important adjuncts to try to minimize damage to the very fragile brain tissue.

FIELD REPORT

An extremely fit, 40-year-old female triathlete from Thailand suddenly complains of an excruciating headache and severe nausea while hiking on a semirural trail. She has never had such a headache before. She rates it a 10/10 on the pain scale. She has no motor signs or symptoms such as one-sided weakness, facial droop, or difficulty speaking. Bystanders lay her down and use spare clothing to insulate her from the bare ground. An ambulance arrives 20 minutes later and takes her to the closest facility with a dedicated stroke team.

Evaluation reveals her to have a congenital brain aneurysm that has started leaking. Emergency angioscopic surgery is performed by the neurosurgery and radiology teams. She makes a full recovery shortly thereafter.

Takeaways

This patient does not fit the classic stroke patient. She is young, fit, does not smoke, and has no underlying health issues. The lessons that should be learned here, along with all other medical and trauma conditions, are as follows: Pay attention to the presenting signs and symptoms of the patient. If they are consistent with a stroke, heart attack, or other condition, assume that's what is happening. Do not disregard possibilities just because the patient does not look like the typical patient in a textbook. Treat their condition as it presents and let the doctors at the hospital decipher the situation more extensively.

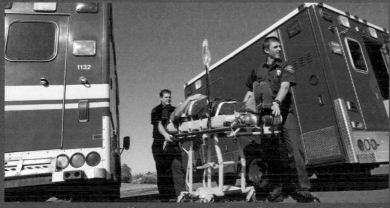

If symptoms suggest a medical emergency, don't wait.
Seek medical care immediately.

SHOCK

The term *shock* is perhaps one of the most overused, misunderstood, and vague words in the medical lexicon. We have all heard that someone "went into shock." Almost no one can accurately define the term. In fact, the word has very little clinical significance, and many, including this author, prefer to use more accurate and specific terminology. It is, however, entrenched in our vocabularies, so a description will be given here.

Technically, the term shock is defined as a combination of tachycardia and cutaneous vasoconstriction. This means that anyone with a fast heart rate and cool, pale skin may be classified as suffering from shock. Obviously, many exceptions to this rule exist. Furthermore, as we will see, some may actually be in a type of shock and exhibit bradycardia (slow heart rate) and cutaneous vasodilation (pink, warm skin). Four basic categories of shock exist.

HYPOVOLEMIC OR HEMORRHAGIC SHOCK

This condition occurs almost exclusively with massive blood loss from either trauma or the sudden rupture of a major blood vessel such as the aorta. A sudden exit of a large quantity of blood from the intravascular space (arteries and veins) results in a variety of immediate compensatory responses. These responses are all evolutionary adaptations designed to maintain the victim's blood pressure. All of our organs depend on blood being delivered to them at a relatively constant pressure. It doesn't matter so much if that pressure comes very often as seen with high heart rates, or more infrequently as with slower rates. To accomplish this requirement of a steady blood pressure, the body uses several regulatory mechanisms. First, the blood vessels that supply the relatively unimportant organs (such as the skin) contract. This is why we see cool, pale skin in individuals who have sustained a massive blood loss event. Second, the heart rate increases. Young, healthy individuals possess a huge capacity to increase their heart rate in the face of such an event. In fact, most people can maintain their blood pressure in the face of ongoing hemorrhage until just before death occurs. The heart rate will increase until it reaches the maximum threshold for that individual. At this point, the compensatory mechanisms are exhausted, and an irreversible death spiral ensues. At this point, the patient is rarely salvageable even with the most advanced, definitive care. The table below demonstrates this in graphic form.

Definitive treatment at a high-level trauma center should obviously be sought immediately for any significant bleeding.

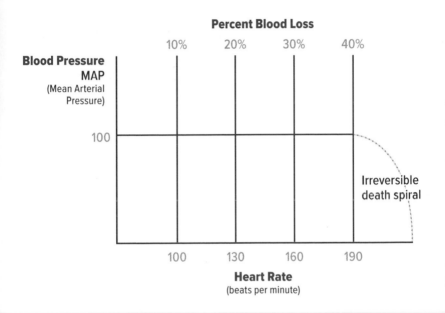

CARDIOGENIC SHOCK

Cardiogenic shock occurs when there is some sort of derangement of the functioning of the heart. Our hearts are nothing more than a cyclic pumping mechanism designed to distribute oxygenated blood to all body tissues and receive deoxygenated (used) blood to be reoxygenated in the lungs to start the cycle anew. Therefore, cardiogenic shock is often referred to as *pump failure.*

This pump failure occurs most commonly in the setting of a heart attack (myocardial infarction). The diagnosis and management of this condition are covered on pages 35–40. To reiterate the salient findings here: chest pain, sweating, nausea, and/or pain in either arm or neck represent common symptoms for an evolving heart attack. The classic shock findings of tachycardia and cutaneous vasoconstriction (pale, cool, clammy skin) are also frequently present.

NEUROGENIC SHOCK

This shock variant is seen after a traumatic transection of the spinal cord at or below the sixth thoracic vertebrae. This sudden loss of all neural signals (both motor and sensory) below this level result in dilation of the blood vessels of the lower extremities and torso with resultant pooling of blood in these locations. This causes a drop in blood pressure. Paradoxically, instead of increasing, the heart rate actually decreases. These two signs represent the *sine quo non* (i.e., nothing else looks like this) of neurogenic shock: hypotension with paradoxical bradycardia. The interesting aspect of this injury is that the patients will frequently complain of minimal or no pain and actually be conversing with rescuers in a relatively normal fashion even though their blood pressure is less than 80.

This injury obviously requires the most expedient evacuation to the nearest trauma center with neurosurgical capabilities. Care should again be taken to meticulously maintain spinal alignment from the skull down to the sacrum.

SEPTIC SHOCK

This type of shock is rarely seen outside of the hospital environment, but it bears mentioning due to the extremely serious nature of the disease. When the body's immune system becomes overwhelmed by microbial infections (most often bacterial), the compensatory mechanisms engage in a last-ditch effort to save the person. The heart rate accelerates dramatically, a high fever typically ensues, and the blood vessels of the skin constrict; nausea and vomiting begin; and finally, the victim becomes delirious before coma and death occur. These individuals may die within a few hours. Definitive medical care must be obtained immediately.

ALTITUDE SICKNESS

The function of the organs in the human body (physiology) occurs within a very limited set of parameters. This includes the height above sea level that we operate in. Between 0 and 5,000 feet above sea level, most folks don't experience any significant issues as it relates to changes in physiology due to altitude. Between 5,000 and 12,000 feet above sea level, those who live at lower elevation and who arrive by car, plane, and other vehicles at these elevations usually experience symptoms due to the relative lack of oxygen at these elevations. Above 12,000 feet, essentially everyone distinctly feels the lower concentration of oxygen.

Many physiological changes occur at altitude. The most obvious ones include faster and deeper respirations to

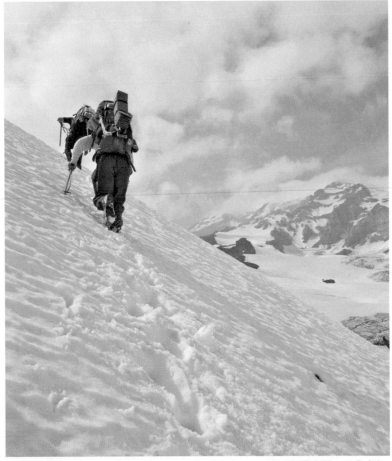

Ascending Mount Rainier

extract more oxygen molecules from an atmosphere that contains fewer of them. Another, more sinister result of rapid elevation gain is that the membranes in the lungs and brain become leaky. This allows fluid to shift from the vascular spaces where it belongs into the tissues of the lungs and brain where it does not. This fluid is not blood but rather the thin, clear fluid devoid of cells that can now pass through these more permeable membranes.

When this fluid passes into the brain tissues, it causes swelling of the brain with significant resultant consequences. This condition is called **HACE—High Altitude Cerebral Edema** (edema just means swelling). When this condition occurs in the lungs, it is called **HAPE—High Altitude Pulmonary Edema.** These conditions may occur separately or together, but for some reason only one of them usually manifests at a time.

These conditions together are sometimes referred to as **AMS—Acute Mountain Sickness.** This is only mentioned for reference, as this term is not particularly specific and therefore of limited use when trying to assess, treat, or relay information to rescue personnel.

HACE and HAPE usually occur when a mountaineer ascends a mountain too quickly and the body does not have sufficient time to adapt to the lower concentration (also called partial pressure) of oxygen along with the lower absolute pressure of the atmosphere. These conditions may occur somewhat randomly at higher elevations even when the climber has adhered to the accepted ascent guidelines. We will now discuss the individual conditions.

HACE

High Altitude Cerebral Edema, as stated above, results from an altitude-related increase in the permeability of the membranous covering of the Central Nervous System. As fluid enters the brain, the resultant swelling puts pressure on the delicate nervous tissue and several very predictable signs and symptoms result. Just as for HAPE and many other conditions, the symptoms are progressive and, if left untreated, may end in the death of the patient. Therefore, the most vital aspect in the management of HACE is early recognition, so that appropriate steps may be taken to halt the process and then to initiate treatment. The signs and symptoms of this condition are listed below.

Early Signs and Symptoms of HACE

- Headache
- Nausea
- Light-headedness
- Fatigue
- Confusion

Late Signs and Symptoms of HACE

- Ataxia (uncoordinated walking, stumbling, falling down)
- Increasingly severe headache
- Increasing confusion
- Diminishing level of consciousness
- Coma
- Death

The progression of HACE is usually very rapid. Left untreated, patients will often die within 24 hours. As the brain swells, it can only push through the opening at the base of the skull (foramen magnum). Unfortunately, the brain is much

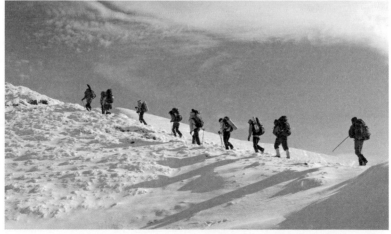

Before you head into the high country, learn to recognize the symptoms of HACE.

too large to fit through this opening and the tissue becomes squished. It is very similar to toothpaste being squeezed out through the top of the tube. Equally unfortunate is that the first brain tissue that contacts the bony opening controls the patient's breathing. As this squeezing occurs, the patient simply stops breathing.

All of this anatomy and physiology information only serves as a backdrop to highlight the importance of extremely rapid recognition and intervention.

Treatment of HACE

The most important treatment for HACE is IMMEDIATE descent. If the condition has been recognized in its latter stages, the patient must be carried or somehow transported to lower elevations. Along with descending, the patient should receive supplemental oxygen and, if available, dexamethasone. Dexamethasone is a steroid preparation that is available in oral or parenteral form (intravenous or intramuscular). Ideally, trained personnel should administer the drug as it is only available in the US by prescription, but if no licensed personnel are available, the drug may be given by nonmedical individuals.

The initial dose is 8–16 mg either orally or through IV, followed by 4 mg every 6 hours thereafter. Obviously, lay personnel should only administer the drug orally.

Treatment should continue until the patient has arrived at an appropriate care facility.

HAPE

The altered physiology responsible for HAPE is the same as for HACE—it just occurs in the lungs instead of the brain. As the leaky membranes allow fluid (interstitial fluid) to enter the lungs, the very thin and delicate air sacs called alveoli rapidly lose their ability to effectively release carbon dioxide and take on oxygen. An interesting anatomy note is that, due to the incredible number of these alveoli, if one were to lay out the surface area of all the alveoli from the lungs of an average adult human it would cover the majority of a football field. Given this incredibly large surface area, it usually takes a bit more time for HAPE to develop into a

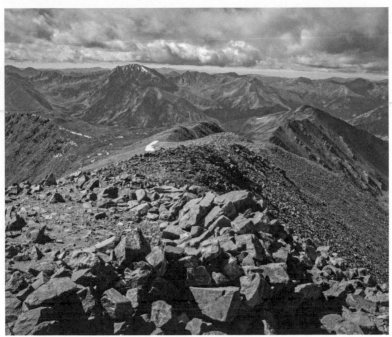
Altitude sickness can occur close to home, too, not just in the Himalayas.

life-threatening problem than for HACE. However, this does not mean that the diagnosis should not be obtained immediately so that treatment may occur. This condition may still kill an individual within 24 hours if not handled appropriately.

The signs and symptoms of HAPE are listed below. The early findings for this condition may mimic those of HACE and are referred to in some writings as Acute Mountain Sickness (AMS).

Early Signs and Symptoms of HAPE
- Headache
- Nausea
- Light-headedness
- Fatigue
- Confusion

Advanced Signs and Symptoms of HAPE
- Blue lips (cyanosis)
- Nonproductive cough (i.e., no sputum is coughed up)

- Dyspnea on exertion (this means the patient experiences more difficulty than normal for a particular exercise)

- Reduced exercise tolerance

Preterminal Signs and Symptoms of HAPE

- Orthopnea (inability to breathe while lying flat)

- Frothy sputum production with cough. This may become pink-tinged as blood vessels burst within the lungs.

- Very high respiratory rate (gasping for air)

- Death

Treatment for HAPE

To reiterate, early recognition is paramount for this condition. The treatment is largely the same as for HACE. IMMEDIATE descent is lifesaving and must be accomplished by whatever means are available. High-flow oxygen and dexamethasone as described for HACE are also indicated. An additional medication called nifedipine is also very helpful for HAPE, but this is not typically available except for well-stocked high-altitude expeditions. If the patient deteriorates to near-death, a breathing tube may be inserted by highly trained individuals and the patient may be mechanically ventilated. These resources should be arranged as soon as the suspicion of a severe case of HAPE is entertained, even if it is not subsequently needed. To call for this help at the last minute would be of no use.

HYPOTHERMIA

As with most medical terms, hypothermia derives from the native language of the earliest modern medical practitioners. In most cases, this means either a Latin or Greek origin. In this case, the Greek *hypo* (under or below) plus *thermé* (heat) form this quite descriptive term.

Within a very narrow range, the human core temperature should be 98.6 degrees Fahrenheit (37 degrees Celsius). Should that core temperature fall below 96 degrees F (36 degrees C), hypothermia occurs. Obviously, the more the internal temperature falls, the more dangerous it is for the individual. Hypothermia may be characterized in terms of severity as follows:

- Mild: 92–96°F
- Moderate: 86–92°F
- Severe: Below 86°F

In a general sense, hypothermia occurs when the environmental conditions overwhelm the body's ability to maintain thermal homeostasis—that is to say, when the insulating capability of the skin and underlying tissues are not sufficiently keeping the cold from penetrating to the deeper, more vital areas. We can think of the situation in a similar way as the insulating capacity of a house. If we fill the exterior walls with insulation, the interior of the house will remain warm. The problem comes when the outside temperature drops low enough so that the insulation is no longer able to prevent the interior temperature from falling.

This problem is exacerbated when moisture enters the equation. The following caveat is critical in the treatment of the hypothermic patient: IT IS IMPOSSIBLE TO WARM A WET, HYPOTHERMIC PATIENT. This point cannot be overstated and will be reiterated in the context of the treatment algorithm outlined below.

Signs and Symptoms of Hypothermia

- Appropriate context (prolonged cold/wet exposure with insufficient protection)
- Shivering
- Pale, cold skin
- Tachycardia (increased heart rate)

As the condition progresses to more advanced stages, the following may be seen:

- Extreme shivering followed by no shivering in the pre-death phase
- Tachycardia transitioning to bradycardia
- Hypotension (low blood pressure)

- Mental status changes (confusion, incoherent speech)
- Paradoxical clothing removal
- Coma/death

All patients suffering from hypothermia must be treated immediately using the following protocol:

- Immediately remove patient from cold/wet environment
- Strip off ALL wet garments and thoroughly dry the patient
- Either redress the patient with warm, dry clothes or place them in a sleeping bag with a rescuer to provide body heat
- Give warm fluids if conscious
- Apply warm water bottles or heat packs to groin/armpits, being careful not to burn the patient
- Descend if at high altitude

Patients who exhibit signs or symptoms of severe hypothermia must be transported immediately to a hospital to receive definitive care. These patients are at risk for developing fatal cardiac arrhythmias (irregular heart rhythms).

FIELD REPORT

A 59-year-old male was descending the standard route on Mount Sneffels in southwest Colorado during a hail/lightning storm. He slipped and sustained a 60-foot tumbling fall. Bystanders reported that the patient was unresponsive and exposed to the storm. They had to evacuate due to extreme lightning danger. The local SAR team responded and, after an hour wait to allow the electrical activity to abate, sent a hasty team to the patient. They found him unresponsive with an obvious head injury and lower extremity injury. He was in the final stages of hypothermia. He exhibited paradoxical clothing removal. Only a faint inguinal pulse was felt. Due to the storm and darkness, evacuation either by litter carry or air asset was not possible. The team quickly stripped the patient, dried him thoroughly, administered supplemental oxygen and placed him in a -20-degree sleeping bag with a chemical heat blanket and warm packs.

Due to the head injury, the patient quickly became combative. He had to be tied to the mountain because he and the entire team were perched on a steep slope. Team members took turns straddling and restraining the patient all night. The entire team was exposed to driving hail and rockfall during the night.

By morning, the patient had normalized his temperature and he began to become coherent and cooperative.

At 7 a.m., a Blackhawk helicopter hoisted the patient off the mountain and into the craft. He was transported to a level 1 trauma center where he made a rapid and full recovery.

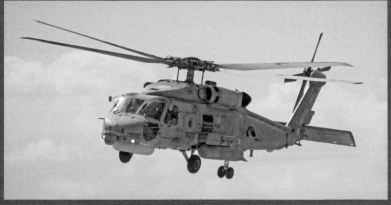

A Blackhawk helicopter used for rescues

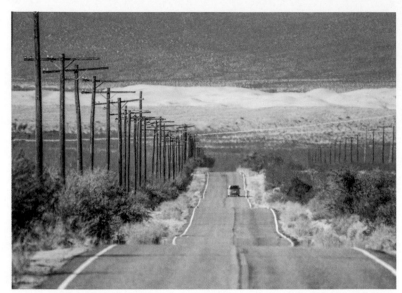
Mojave National Preserve, California; when you're outside in the heat, be aware of overheating.

HYPERTHERMIA

By exactly the same mechanism, hyperthermia (*hyper*—over; *thermé*—heat) results when the skin and other compensatory mechanisms become overwhelmed by a too-hot environment. Any time an individual ventures outdoors when the ambient temperature exceeds that of the body's core temperature (98.6 degrees F), they are at risk for the development of hyperthermia. Exertion at such temperatures markedly exacerbates that risk.

Note that the term hyperthermia has replaced the old *heat stroke* and *heat exhaustion*, which are not accurate nor appropriately descriptive terms.

We have all been hot while recreating in the backcountry, and so the distinction between acceptable functioning in a hot environment and hyperthermia becomes both difficult and imperative to determine. In order to maintain the narrow range of acceptable core temperatures as mentioned in the section describing hypothermia, the body employs cooling mechanisms when faced with the possibility of overheating. First, sweating occurs to take advantage of the so-called "latent heat of evaporation." When water evaporates, it creates a cooling effect on the surface that it's in contact with. In the case of humans, that surface is the skin.

The higher our core temperature rises, the more we sweat. Our breathing rate also increases in an attempt to dissipate heat in the form of water vapor from our lungs.

Unfortunately, as with all compensatory mechanisms, there are limits. When we begin to run out of bodily fluids to sweat out and expel from the lungs, the early stages of hyperthermia set in. We lose the ability to sweat, which markedly diminishes the capacity to cool ourselves. After this occurs, the core temperature rises rapidly, resulting very quickly in irreversible organ failure and death. This vicious downward cycle may be fatal in a shockingly short period of time—less than an hour in extreme cases. Therefore, early and aggressive treatment will be lifesaving for this dangerous condition.

Signs and Symptoms of Mild Hyperthermia

- Sweating
- Rapid respirations
- Thirst

Signs and Symptoms of Moderate to Severe Hyperthermia

- Excessive sweating followed by complete absence of sweating
- Very rapid respirations
- Extreme thirst
- Diminished urine output (very dark-colored urine) followed by absence of urine output
- Confusion followed by decreased level of consciousness
- Coma and death

Treatment Should Be Immediate and Aggressive

- Removal from sun or hot environment
- Immersion in cool (not icy cold) water if possible
- Wetting entire skin surface area with water if immersion is not possible
- Cold water/electrolyte solution if conscious

- Ice packs to groin/axilla
- Immediate transport to hospital for moderate–severe cases, as fatal cardiac arrhythmias and/or organ failure may result

FROSTBITE AND CHILBLAINS

Frostbite represents a serious condition in which inadequately protected tissue freezes and dies when exposed to outside temperatures low enough to overcome the body's natural thermal barriers. The torso represents the thermal core; therefore, the tissues farthest away from this heat source are at the highest risk for freezing. These vulnerable areas include toes, fingers, nose, and cheeks. More extreme and/or prolonged exposure to freezing conditions will put additional tissues such as feet and hands at risk.

As with all injury processes, prevention remains the most effective tool in the kit. High-altitude mountaineers are especially prone to the development of frostbite. It becomes imperative, therefore, that upon ascending, frequent reassessments of clothing such as gloves/mittens and overboots be performed. Frequent checks of at-risk tissue such as fingers and faces should be considered as well. At times, the effort of ascending a mountain at high elevations, especially above 20,000 feet, may be all-encompassing and an individual may forget these important checks. Also, the temperature essentially always decreases with increasing elevation. The alpinist must be cognizant of this fact and add layers as needed. Individuals should descend immediately at any sign of freezing tissue.

DIAGNOSIS

The diagnosis of frostbite is relatively straightforward. The small blood vessels (capillaries) freeze first. This sudden lack of blood flow causes a blanching effect and the tissues appear pale. Without immediate treatment, the tissues that are supplied with oxygen and nutrients via these small blood vessels begin to die. This process is called necrosis. When this occurs, the skin starts to turn blue and blister (Figure 1). This phase indicates that the affected tissue is actively dying, and some of it may actually be nonviable at this point. As the condition progresses, irreversible damage occurs and the tissue turns black (Figure 2). At this point, the black tissue is beyond repair and will require amputation at some point in the future.

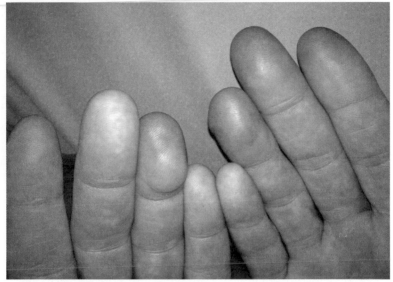

Figure 1

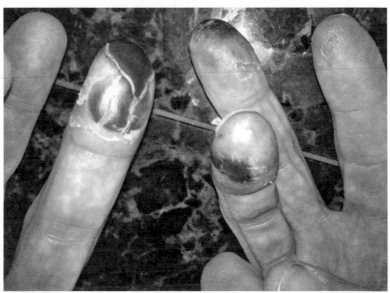

Figure 2
Frostbite, untreated, can lead to tissue loss (and necessitate amputation).

TREATMENT

Treatment for this very serious condition requires rapid recognition and the completion of a series of specific maneuvers.

1) The patient must be immediately removed from the freezing environment. This may include establishing a hasty campsite high on a mountain. Ideally, a patient who is experiencing frostbite in a high altitude should descend with the utmost haste. This will accomplish two objectives. First, the temperature usually increases as the elevation decreases. Second, the concentration of oxygen increases at lower elevations. This gas is imperative in order to preserve as much tissue as possible. It is also important to dry the affected areas immediately. Wet skin cannot be effectively warmed. These three considerations—protection from the environment, drying, and descent—are all integral parts of the immediate treatment algorithm. The exact order of their performance depends on the individual circumstance, but they should all be accomplished as soon as possible.

2) Immediate rewarming with moist heat. Several critical points should be made here. First, the tissues must not be warmed and then allowed to refreeze. This will compound the amount of irreversible tissue damage. Frostbite always involves at least some tissue that has sustained serious but survivable damage. This transition zone between dead tissue and live tissue represents our target for treatment. Tissue that has already passed into the nonrecoverable stage will not be affected by treatment. It is the live tissue and the tissue that is in the process of asphyxiation that must be protected. The exposed tissue is ideally placed in warm, not hot, water. The temperature of the water should be roughly that of a hot tub: 102–106 degrees Fahrenheit. Water hotter than this may burn the tissue, and water cooler than this may not effectively rewarm the cells that are struggling to stay alive. This may be continued for 20 minutes or so and repeated as the situation permits. As soon as the affected part is out of the water, it must be immediately dried and placed inside a warm garment.

3) Supplemental oxygen. As mentioned previously, all human cells require oxygen in order to function. Especially at elevation, giving additional oxygen to the patient via a nasal cannula will aid in the optimization of the healing environment.

4) Immediate definitive medical care must be sought.

DIABETES

Without delving too deeply into the biochemistry of diabetes, we will provide a general description of what diabetes means, as well as the field recognition of symptoms associated with this disease process along with backcountry treatment algorithms.

The term diabetes refers to conditions in which the body is unable to process carbohydrates (sugars) properly. The defect arises from an altered metabolism of the hormone called insulin. Insulin is produced by the pancreas and is essential for the proper utilization of glucose by cells all over the body. Glucose is the carbohydrate most frequently used by the body to power activities ranging from muscular contractions to higher thought processes. Insulin functions as a sort of escort for glucose to pass through cell membranes and thus be available as a fuel source. When this process breaks down, not only does the fuel supply for cellular functions diminish, but the buildup of glucose in the bloodstream produces a potentially life-threatening situation.

Two basic forms of diabetes exist.

Type 1 diabetes is caused by the body attacking the cells that produce insulin in the pancreas. This autoimmune assault typically occurs during childhood and requires that

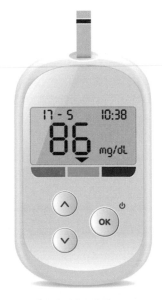

Monitoring blood sugar levels is essential for those with diabetes.

the affected individual receive daily insulin administration and careful measurement of blood glucose levels to survive.

Type 2 diabetes represents 90–95% of the cases of this disease in the United States and is directly attributable to unhealthy lifestyle choices. These choices primarily include lifelong consumption of highly processed carbohydrates. Our bodies have not adapted evolutionarily to the utilization of such large quantities of these very concentrated sugars, so our cells become resistant to the actions of insulin on the cell membranes. This helps prevent the buildup of glucose within the cells, but the consequence is that this sugar builds up within the bloodstream. Over time, this excess sugar causes end-organ damage to the brain, eyes, heart, kidneys, and liver.

While both types of diabetes may produce organ dysfunction and early death over time, in the backcountry we are only worried about the immediate effects of serum blood sugars that are either too high or too low.

ASSESSMENT OF POSSIBLE DIABETES COMPLICATIONS

As with all other medical conditions, a careful history and a high index of suspicion are essential to the most accurate identification of diabetic issues. First, the patient should be questioned regarding their current symptoms, daily blood sugar measuring regimen, and insulin and/or diabetic medication administration schedule. If the patient is unable to provide this information, a companion with knowledge of the patient's situation should be interrogated. If no such person is available, the rescuer must rely on the patient's signs/symptoms along with blood sugar measuring equipment when it becomes available.

If patients are coherent, they can usually tell if their blood glucose is too high or too low. Just that information alone can be enough to initiate field treatment even before glucometers (blood glucose measuring devices) are available.

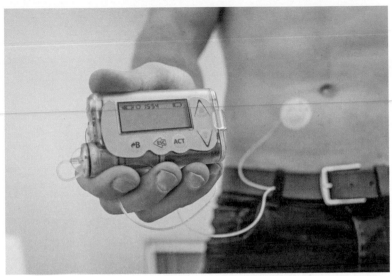
An insulin pump for type 1 diabetes

TYPE 1 DIABETES

It should be noted that juvenile onset or type 1 diabetics are especially prone to rapid and unpredictable swings in their blood sugar. These patients will frequently be wearing an insulin pump. This pump is essentially a reservoir of liquid insulin in a disc-shaped case that is attached to the skin, usually near the waist. A small, clear tube extends from the reservoir to a needle inserted under the skin. A separate sensor on the device measures the blood sugar levels and automatically administers a preset dose of insulin.

Various problems may occur with this device. The reservoir may run dry, the sensor may malfunction, the patient may consume a very large quantity of high-glycemic carbohydrates that temporarily overwhelms the system, or the patient may not eat enough food for the dose of insulin supplied and the blood sugar may drop too low. Regardless of the problem, the device should be inspected to the best of the rescuers' capability. Care must be taken not to dislodge the device from the patient's skin during the inspection process. If the rescuer does not feel comfortable looking at the device, it is best left alone.

Below are listed signs and symptoms manifested by patients whose blood sugar is too low (hypoglycemia) or too high (hyperglycemia).

Hypoglycemia (Low Blood Sugar)

- Pale
- Sweating
- Shakiness
- Irregular/fast heartbeat
- Hunger
- Irritability/change in mood
- Fatigue
- Headache
- Nausea

Severe, Potentially Life-threatening Hypoglycemia

- Diminished wakefulness/level of consciousness
- Coma
- Death

Hyperglycemia (High Blood Sugar)

- Frequent urination
- Thirst (may be extreme)
- Blurred vision
- Numbness and/or tingling in hands and feet

It should be obvious that many of the above symptoms may be seen with other medical conditions; therefore, a detailed history and situational awareness of the patient's condition are paramount in accurately assessing the situation.

FIELD TREATMENT

Regardless of whether the patient is experiencing a hypo- or hyperglycemic event, a glucometer should be obtained as quickly as possible to verify the diagnosis and to monitor the glucose levels during the first few hours of treatment. If this is not immediately available, the rescuer should use the above lists of signs and symptoms to determine the patient's suspected glucose abnormality. Treatment is as follows.

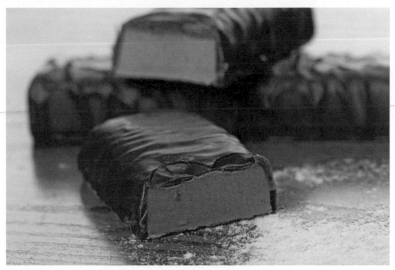
In the case of low blood sugar, sugary drinks or energy bars are a good option.

Hypoglycemia

Administer high-sugar liquid such as orange juice or other sugary drinks. If the patient is able to swallow, these drinks should be followed by a small protein meal such as a protein-containing energy bar, nuts, peanut butter, etc. As the patient recovers, the rescuer may more fully flesh out the recent history to ascertain if the patient received too much insulin, didn't eat enough, or some other factor is at play. No further treatment is required once the patient fully recovers.

Hyperglycemia

Known diabetics will regularly receive either insulin or oral medication such as metformin, or both. If the patient is conscious, they can direct the administration of the correct medications. Licensed medical personnel may also do this. Lay persons should receive direction from trained clinicians before administering any medication. The patient must also stay hydrated with water and/or non-sugar-containing electrolyte solutions.

If the patient is unconscious, the urgency of the situation rises dramatically, and the victim should generally be transported by air to the nearest hospital, attended by paramedics or similarly trained individuals who can place an IV, administer medications, and more.

SEIZURES

The topic of seizures represents a very broad set of considerations. We will focus only on the issues germane to backcountry management of this condition.

The term seizure indicates a situation where a spot in the brain engages in uncontrolled, random discharges of neurons. This event then produces violent, involuntary muscle spasms. The scope of these spasms can be anywhere from imperceptible muscle twitches and a mild decreased level of consciousness to total body spasmodic contractions and complete loss of consciousness. This latter group is generally referred to as *grand mal* or, in medical terms, *generalized tonic-clonic* seizures.

Often, individuals know beforehand that they suffer from this episodic condition and take daily medication for it. If patients forget their medication or take other substances such as new medications that interfere with the absorption of the anti-seizure medication, they may be more prone to such an attack. Unfortunately, absent a hospital setting, not much can be done in the backcountry to stop the event once it has begun. Our job as rescuers is to attempt to mitigate the negative effects of such an occurrence. Some of these negative effects include: airway obstruction due to tongue falling back into throat or blood/teeth if the patient bites their tongue or breaks a tooth, inability to generate adequate respiratory effort if the seizure lasts long enough, and trauma from falling to the ground or off of a high place.

To ameliorate these potentially untoward results, the rescuer(s) should do the following:

- Lay the patient on their side in a safe place. The patient may vomit, so side positioning is very important to prevent aspiration into the airways.

- If possible, position an object between the teeth, such as part of a towel, to allow ingress for air and to prevent the person from biting the tongue or breaking teeth.

- Do not place fingers into the mouth—they will be bitten!

- Consider calling for assistance if trauma has occurred or the seizure lasts more than 30 seconds or so.

After the event has passed, the person should ideally be removed from the remote setting to obtain an assessment from a neurologist. Seizures can frequently reoccur, especially if the patient's medication needs to be readjusted.

ASTHMA

Asthma is the word we use for any condition in which an environmental agent (antigen in medical parlance) causes a sudden constriction of the airways. We call these situations asthma attacks. The more accurate term is *Reactive Airway Disease.* Such episodes can range from a bit unsettling to lethal. Thousands of individuals die each year from asthma attacks, so we must take each one very seriously.

More often than not, people have suffered from asthma for years and are quite aware of the triggering agents. If they are new to the backcountry, however, they may encounter pollen or other particles that they have not been exposed to before. Such new antigens may bring on an attack in a susceptible individual. Asthma sufferers usually carry an inhaler to use at the first sign of an attack. Typically, this inhaler contains a medication that opens up constricted air passages (a bronchodilator).

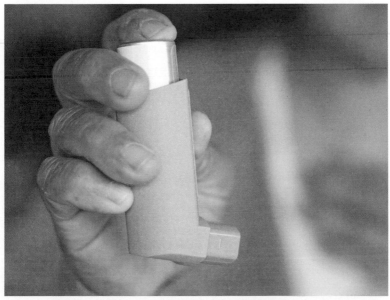

Asthma sufferers should always bring along their prescribed inhalers.

OPIOID OVERDOSE

Although not traditionally within the purview of backcountry medicine topics, the incidence of drug overdoses in the United States has escalated to epidemic proportions. Opioid medications such as **morphine, fentanyl,** and **oxycodone** were once only available in hospital settings or by closely regulated prescriptions. Due to the thriving illicit drug trade, both within and outside our borders, these drugs are now widely available for recreational use.

These drugs are all highly addictive as well as dangerous. The term used to describe those addicted to such medications is **Opioid Use Disorder (OUD).**

Addicts seek out these drugs for the properties of euphoria and pain relief (analgesia). Unfortunately, these outwardly positive attributes come at a cost. The side effects listed below can be, and frequently are, deadly.

Opioid Side Effects

- Disorientation
- Agitation/violent tendencies
- Somnolence
- Coma
- Death

Death occurs when a victim overdoses, and the drug depresses the respiratory center in the brain leading to respiratory failure. Death can occur within a few minutes.

Signs and Symptoms of Opioid Overdose

- Small (constricted) pupils
- Diminished level of consciousness and responsiveness
- Shallow, slow breathing
- Progression to no breathing at all

These findings should be interpreted in the appropriate clinical context to distinguish between other conditions. It should be reiterated that one of the most tell-tale findings is small, equal pupils in the setting of respiratory depression. Ascertaining that the patient has suffered from OUD or has had a witnessed ingestion of an opioid by a bystander is very helpful.

Treatment should be rapid and decisive. An antidote for opioid overdose exists—**naloxone**. The brand name is **Narcan**. Naloxone works by rapidly reversing the effects of opioids. Two delivery methods exist: nasal inhalation and injectable. Both forms are available at most pharmacies without a prescription. Nasal inhalation is far and away the easiest method of delivery for non–medically trained individuals. Unfortunately, this method requires a marginally cooperative patient. Those who have passed into unconsciousness are better served with the injectable form, but the nasal administration should be used if that is what is available. Several doses may be required, as sometimes a relapse occurs if the patient has ingested an exceptionally large quantity of the drug.

A very useful tool is the CDC (Centers for Disease Control) website: cdc.gov. A free training module of excellent quality is available. Anyone who thinks they may have occasion to respond to such an emergency should watch it. Similarly, consider carrying Narcan in your first aid kit—either in the car, home, or backcountry—depending on the potential for deployment.

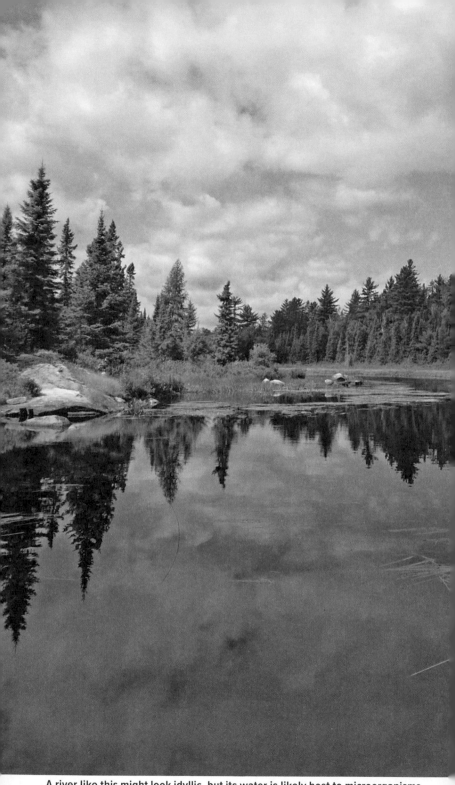

A river like this might look idyllic, but its water is likely host to microorganisms that can make you sick, making water purification essential. (See pages 86–87.)

Just as in the urban setting, a staggering array of infectious possibilities exist in the backcountry. The difference here is that help is much farther away, so prompt recognition and early treatment become even more important. In this chapter, we will divide infections into categories depending upon the body part or organ system involved. The unifying element in all of these is that they are caused by a microscopic organism of some sort. The variety of organisms far surpasses the capacity of a single text to delineate. Our purpose here is to provide a potential rescuer with the knowledge to recognize the fact that an infection has taken place, then outline steps that may be taken in a backcountry setting to ameliorate the process. We will break down these infections into broad categories. Although some specific responsible organisms will be mentioned, it is not necessary to compile an exhaustive list of bacteria, viruses, spirochetes, and more.

CENTRAL NERVOUS SYSTEM INFECTIONS

The central nervous system (CNS) is composed of the brain and spinal cord. Protecting these vital structures are three separate membrane layers collectively called meninges. When an infection affects these layers, a condition called meningitis occurs. It is no surprise that an infection of these tissues represents a severe and potentially life-threatening situation. An infectious process that involves the meninges may be fatal in only a few hours. Therefore, it is vitally important that this condition be recognized immediately by a rescuer in the backcountry so that early evacuation and treatment may be instituted.

MENINGITIS

Meningitis may result from either viruses or bacteria, although bacterial meningitis represents the most common condition. Generally, bacteria infect the meninges by traversing this bony plate inside the nose that separates the mid-face from the brain. Children are particularly susceptible to bacterial meningitis. Seemingly insignificant head trauma may allow bacteria to enter the CNS spaces and cause this condition. Alternatively, viruses or bacteria may precipitate this infectious process without any recognizable antecedent event.

Signs and Symptoms of Meningitis

- Headache (usually severe)
- Stiff neck, painful on flexion (chin to chest); this condition is called meningismus and is diagnostic of meningitis
- Pain in eyes on exposure to sunlight or bright lights (photophobia)
- Fever—may be very high, especially in children
- Skin rash—not one of the more common signs

Signs and Symptoms of Severe/Advanced Meningitis

- Drowsiness/altered level of consciousness
- Seizures
- Coma
- Death

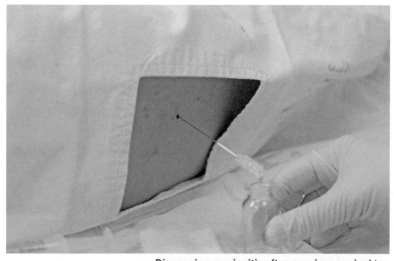

Diagnosing meningitis often requires a spinal tap

Again, time is of the essence here. Not much can be done in the field as far as treatment. The diagnosis must be made rapidly and definitively. The patient must be flown to a hospital immediately. Any patient who exhibits the majority of the above symptoms should be considered to have acute meningitis. Even if this proves not to be the case after arrival at a hospital, there is no way to determine this in the field. It is okay if the patient turns out to not have meningitis and only experiences a helicopter ride. It is not okay if the diagnosis is not considered and the patient dies.

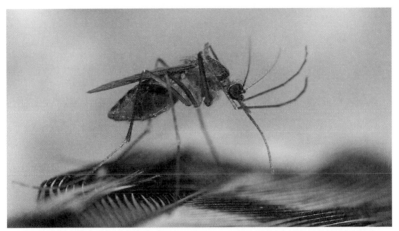

Mosquitoes are common carriers of encephalitis.
Credit: CDC/The Connecticut Agricultural Experiment Station

ENCEPHALITIS

Lying underneath the meninges are the brain and spinal cord. These obviously critical structures may also be infected with viruses and bacteria after all other lines of defense (skin, soft tissues, bones, meninges) have been breached. Unfortunately, the CNS is composed of tissues that represent an extremely fertile environment for foreign invaders. This means that infections here rapidly become fatal if not treated within a few hours.

Mosquitoes and ticks carry several viruses that produce encephalitis. This is another reason that protection from insect bites becomes so important. Bacteria, fungi, and other organisms may also cause encephalitis, but these agents are distinctly rarer, and the onset of the disease process is usually over days to weeks instead of hours.

As with meningitis, no effective field treatment exists for encephalitis. The rescuer must identify the condition and arrange for expeditious evacuation.

Signs and Symptoms of Encephalitis

- Headache (usually severe)
- Stiff neck (meningismus)
- Pain on exposure to light (photophobia)
- Fever—usually high (102 degrees F and above)
- Sensitivity to sound
- Involuntary movements

Signs and Symptoms of Severe/Advanced Encephalitis

- Confusion, agitation, and even hallucinations
- Loss of motor function in certain parts of the body (may be difficult to distinguish from stroke)
- Muscle weakness
- Difficulty hearing
- Abnormal speech or unable to speak (aphasias)
- Seizures
- Diminished level of consciousness
- Coma
- Death

Note that many of the signs and symptoms of encephalitis are the same as for meningitis. Many are even typical for stroke victims. The real takeaway here is that the rescuer does not have to have a medical degree nor be able to accurately make a perfect diagnosis. The presence of essentially any of the above severe signs and/or symptoms warrants immediate evacuation. It is fine if the rescuer reports to the 911 dispatcher, for instance, that the patient is suffering from some or all of the above signs and symptoms and says, "I don't know if this is meningitis, encephalitis, or stroke." The field protocol is the same—immediate evacuation.

PULMONARY INFECTIONS

At rest, adult humans typically breathe 12–20 times per minute, making the lungs uniquely positioned for significant environmental exposure. This means that any pathogen in the air may be inhaled and thus incorporated into the body. In a normal state of immunocompetency (i.e., no underlying conditions that would weaken the immune system), the lungs possess a tremendous capacity to neutralize potential invaders. This is not always the case, however. Other factors that can influence whether the body can fight off airborne invaders include state of nutrition, physical exhaustion, altitude, and a higher-than-normal concentration of environmental exposure. Some densely populated cities, for instance, cause increased numbers of pulmonary infections due to higher concentrations of airborne viruses and bacteria coupled with high levels of pollutants that may weaken the immune system. An example would be travelers passing through Kathmandu on their way to a Himalayan expedition. It is very common for expedition members to acquire

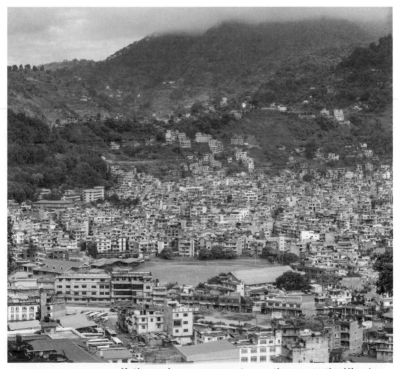

Kathmandu, a common stop on the way to the Himalayas

some sort of lung infection in this Nepalese capital, then travel to high altitudes where their bodies are less able to combat the infection.

PREVENTION OF PULMONARY INFECTIONS

The primary prevention for pulmonary infection includes avoidance of close contact with potentially infected individuals. This means not sharing indoor spaces and maintaining a 6–10-foot spacing in the outdoors with those individuals.

At the time of this writing, the COVID-19 pandemic is stretching into its third year. High-quality masks that filter airborne particulates and droplets represent excellent defense adjuncts for this and other viruses when used properly (fitting the face and covering both mouth and nose). Note that viruses may enter the body through the eyes as well as the nose and mouth. Therefore, wraparound eye protection is essential in high-risk situations.

Vaccines are available for this novel viral disease and should be received at the direction of the CDC. As with all viruses, this particular coronavirus mutates constantly, requiring revaccination periodically just as for the influenza virus.

PULMONARY INFECTIONS CAUSED BY VIRUSES

As mentioned above, the causative virus for COVID-19 is an extremely easily transmitted pathogen. The fact is that most viruses, such as the SARS-CoV and avian flu viruses, have caused either epidemics (diseases confined to a single

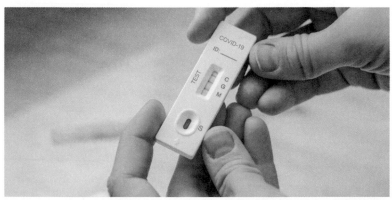

An over-the-counter COVID test

population) or pandemics (diseases that have traversed countries or population groups) in the past and are always a threat to reemerge. They are all quite easily transmitted human-to-human through airborne contact. The incubation period for these viruses typically ranges from 2 to 7 days. This period is the time that passes from initial exposure until the patient experiences symptoms. Unfortunately, patients are typically capable of spreading the disease before they manifest significant symptoms. This fact is one of the many reasons that respiratory viruses are such successful invaders.

Signs and Symptoms of Common Respiratory Viral Infections

- Chest or nasal congestion
- Wet or dry cough
- Runny nose
- Fatigue
- Body aches
- Low-grade fever
- Sore throat

Infections that progress to cause deeper lung infections (viral pneumonias) are much more serious. Signs and symptoms that this has occurred include:

- Persistent, hacking cough
- Markedly increased respiratory rate (20–40 breaths/minute)
- High fevers

Most viral infections are self-limiting. Treatment includes rest, fluids, and antipyretics (fever reducers) such as ibuprofen and acetaminophen. Those with more serious infections and those whose clinical condition worsens should be evacuated.

Children, and especially infants, with respiratory symptoms should receive medical care from their doctor as soon as possible.

PULMONARY INFECTIONS CAUSED BY BACTERIA

Bacteria may cause respiratory infections in the same way that viruses do—by passing into the pulmonary tissues with inhalation. In contrast to viral infections, however, bacterial infections often produce more pronounced symptoms, such as a cough productive of greenish or yellowish sputum. They are also treatable with antibiotics. As of this writing, there are no specific virucidal (virus-killing) agents. Bacteria may infect the respiratory system anywhere from the nasal passages to the deep recesses of the chest cavity. Specific sites of infection, along with their signs and symptoms, are listed below.

Sinus Infections

- Headache

- Fever

- Pain with gentle finger tapping over sinuses (cheeks, forehead)

Pharyngitis (infection of the throat)

- Sore throat

- Fever

- Yellowish and/or whitish coating of the back of the throat (exudative pharyngitis)

- Cough

Tracheitis (infection of the main airway)

- Painful respirations deep in the chest

- Fever

- Cough

- Labored, painful breathing

Pneumonia

- Cough; usually producing yellowish sputum (productive cough)
- Fever
- Chills
- Malaise
- Rapid, shallow breathing
- Pain with deep inhalation

Although any of the above conditions may progress to a serious, even life-threatening situation, the last category, bacterial pneumonia, represents the most consistently dangerous condition. All of the above will typically require a course of antibiotic therapy to cure, but pneumonia often requires hospitalization with intravenous antibiotics.

Field treatment for all of the above infections consists of rest, fluids, ibuprofen and/or acetaminophen, and antibiotics. Antibiotics should only be administered after a physician examination, except under unusual circumstances such as serious infections in the setting of delayed evacuation.

FIELD REPORT

A mixed group of Americans and Britons join to form an expedition with the goal of climbing Ama Dablam, a 22,500-foot mountain adjacent to Mount Everest (Chomolungma) in Nepal. During the multiday acclimatization trek into the region, one of the team members begins to cough. Over the next several days, the cough becomes more severe until it becomes an almost constant series of violent spasmodic expectorations. At basecamp, he is bed-ridden for several days under the care of the medical team. He receives antibiotics and cough suppressants. After 5–6 days, he has improved enough to allow himself to walk around base-camp. Unfortunately, he has missed his climbing window and is unable to attempt to ascend the mountain. Instead, he faces a long march back to civilization along with the successful summiteers.

The salient point here is that one should be aware of one's sur-roundings, including hazards unique to the travel zone. In Nepal, the extremely busy main trail systems are utilized not only by humans, but also by domesticated animals such as yaks, naks, and zupyuks. The animals urinate and defecate on the trails. These excretions mix with the very fine dust that composes the soil of the high pla-teaus. This dust can easily enter the lungs of trekkers, along with a very high concentration of bacteria, viruses, and parasites. This is the reason for the high incidence of pulmonary infections, including severe pneumonias, which afflict travelers in this region.

Understanding this issue beforehand and taking adequate pre-cautions, such as wearing masks or buffs, hiking at night during lower use times, and choosing lesser-traveled routes, might have prevented the infection in this individual.

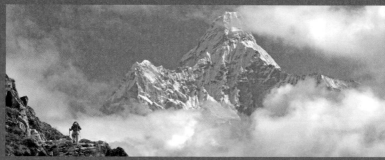

Ama Dablam in the Himalayas

GASTROINTESTINAL INFECTIONS

Given the constant interaction between the gastrointestinal system and the environment by way of ingesting food and liquids, it's no surprise that, especially in the backcountry, pathogens (bacteria, viruses, parasites) frequently enter the intestinal tract and cause infections. The number of organisms with the potential to cause these infections are legion. In the backcountry, identifying the causative organism is not nearly as important as the early implementation of a treatment program to limit the ramifications of the infection. If necessary, detailed analysis of the patient's stool and/or blood may be performed at a tertiary care facility to pinpoint the diagnosis and precisely determine the correct treatment regimen. As the resources available are typically severely limited in rural environments, the treatment algorithms are largely the same irrespective of the causative organism.

The signs and symptoms of gastrointestinal infections may be broken down into foregut (mouth, esophagus, stomach, and the beginning of the small intestine) and hindgut (most of the small intestines and large intestine) symptoms.

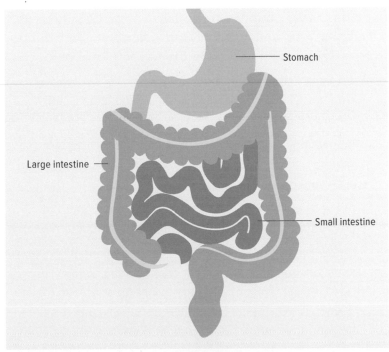

Stomach

Large intestine

Small intestine

A simplified look at the gastrointestinal system

Signs and Symptoms of Foregut Infections

- Nausea
- Vomiting
- Stomach cramps
- Sweating
- Fever

Again, these infections may be caused by viruses, bacteria, or parasites. Due to the chemical makeup of the fluid within the foregut, viruses are more commonly involved in this location.

Signs and Symptoms of Hindgut Infections

- Nausea
- Vomiting
- Diarrhea, including bloody diarrhea
- Lower abdominal cramping
- Fever

Note that infections of any part of the GI system may produce severe dehydration and electrolyte imbalances, especially in infants and children. Therefore, immediate treatment should be instituted. This treatment includes:

- Oral fluids including electrolytes (sodium, potassium, possibly magnesium)
- Intravenous fluids for severely ill individuals. This will require transport out of the backcountry to a center where such care is available..
- Antinausea medications (Phenergan, Zofran, etc.; administered by licensed personnel)
- Antibiotics. Note that the administration of antibiotics for GI infections remains somewhat controversial. Some clinicians recommend allowing these infections to "run their course." Given the fact that there is no way to determine the causative agent for these infections in the backcountry, most professionals who deal with backcountry medicine

recommend a trial of antibiotics, if available, for patients with moderate to severe symptoms. Although all medications have potential side effects, antibiotics represent a class of medications with a very low side-effect profile, with the exception of patients who are allergic to a specific antibiotic. Therefore, it is critical for the patient to be carefully questioned regarding any antibiotic allergies.

Also, as stated above, hindgut infections (traveler's diarrhea, etc.) are more likely to be caused by organisms susceptible to antibiotics (bacteria such as Giardia, parasites). These patients also do not present with nausea as a primary symptom as a rule, which allows them to be able to keep down the antibiotics more frequently.

Currently there's no consensus among researchers regarding the optimal antibiotic regimen for backcountry intestinal infections. As of this writing, Azithromycin (trade name Z-pak when it comes prepackaged as a five-day course) represents the most commonly prescribed antibiotic for this condition. The typical course is 500 milligrams (mg) the first day followed by 250 mg for the subsequent four days.

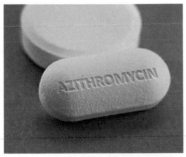

As always, all medications come with potential side effects, so ideally the antibiotics should be given under the advice of a physician.

Azithromycin is a common treatment prescribed for backcountry intestinal ailments.

If the infection persists or worsens despite the antibiotic treatment, seek definitive medical care.

GI INFECTION PREVENTION

Obviously, prevention of any infection represents the best form of therapy. To this end, meticulous personal hygiene is the cornerstone of GI tract infection prevention. After urination or defecation, wash hands with soap and water for at least 10 seconds. Pay special attention to the hand that is involved in wiping the anus or genitalia. Alcohol-based antimicrobial gels are also very effective for killing disease-causing

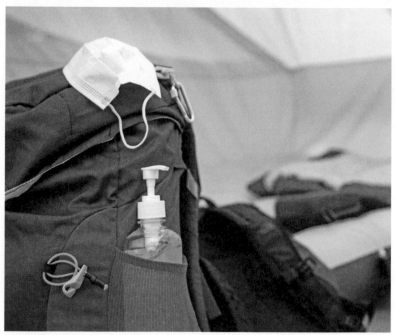
Alcohol-based hand sanitizer is a good choice for backcountry hand hygiene.

organisms on the hands. In fact, these alcohol preparations kill the vast majority of bacteria and viruses. There are several notable exceptions, however, so the ideal regimen includes a thorough handwashing followed by drying and then the application of an alcohol gel, which is worked onto all fingers. These tenets become especially germane when folks are sharing food or drinks.

Water purification in the backcountry is similarly essential in the prevention of ingested pathogens. A large array of microorganisms, including *Giardia lamblia,* cryptosporidium, and many others, are lurking in roughly 99% of the waterways in the US. Therefore, purifying water before drinking it is a vital step to ensuring a disease-free wilderness experience. You may purify water in four basic ways.

1. Boiling   This is the oldest purification method. Due to the decreased atmospheric pressure at higher elevations, water will require additional boiling time to achieve full purification. This is because the higher we climb, the lower the boiling point of water. At sea level, water boils at 212°F. At 10,000 feet above sea level, the boiling point is 194°F. Basically, this translates to

1 minute of a full boil below 5,000 feet in elevation and up to 3–4 minutes at higher elevations. The exact time depends on the elevation. At 20,000 feet 4 minutes may be required, while at 10,000 feet 2 minutes may be sufficient. Appropriate boiling kills all potential pathogens.

2. Chemical purification This has traditionally meant iodine tablets. While these tablets are effective, they turn all water containers brown and impart a mildly disagreeable taste to the water. Chlorine and bromine tablets/ liquids are also available and just as effective. They don't give such an unpleasant taste to the water either. All of these chemicals are effective in producing safe drinking water as long as the directions are followed. This typically means allowing the substance to dissolve completely in the water, shaking the container vigorously, and then waiting at least 20 minutes before drinking. Longer waits are necessary for colder water.

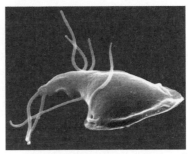
An electron microscope image of *Giardia lamblia*

3. Filters Water filters have been around for decades. They basically consist of a cylinder containing a series of filters through which water is forcefully pumped. These fine filters remove the pathogens from the water. They produce excellent-quality drinking water. The downsides are that they are heavy and the filters must be changed fairly frequently.

4. UV light As of the last 10 years or so, UV pens have become available. These devices are inserted into a container of water (usually 1 liter maximum) and agitated for the time recommended by the manufacturer. These products work fairly well, but likely not as well as the methods mentioned above, and less so in water with a large particle count. They also require the user to carry batteries and extra UV bulbs.

APPENDICITIS

Although a number of surgical emergencies may afflict the abdominal cavity, one in particular merits special attention: appendicitis. Appendicitis is the term applied to the condition in which the appendix becomes inflamed. This almost always occurs when the inside of the hollow appendix becomes blocked by a hard piece of stool. This obstruction is called a fecolith. To better understand what happens, we will briefly look at the anatomy of this vestigial organ (it doesn't serve any current purpose but likely did in the remote past).

The appendix is nothing more than a hollow tube open to the inside of the colon and closed at the other end.

When this tube becomes blocked, the portion of the appendix beyond the blockage swells. Because it is part of the colon, which is teeming with bacteria, infection sets in quickly. If surgical intervention is not completed quickly, the organ may rupture. This process will spill stool and bacteria into the abdominal cavity, which will result in a condition called peritonitis. This can cause death within only a day or two if left untreated.

The diagnosis of appendicitis is often quite straightforward. The caveat here is that this disease process is often referred to as the "great imitator" due to the sometimes unusual constellation of presenting signs and symptoms.

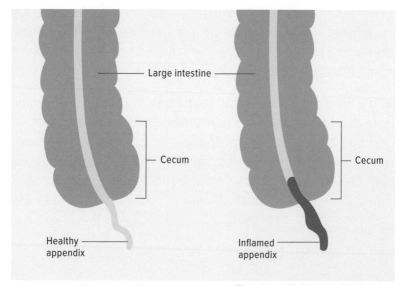

The appendix is part of the colon.

Without delving too deep into the nuances of this process, the usual signs and symptoms are listed below.

Early appendicitis (0–12 hours)

- Anorexia. This is the medical term for not feeling hungry and is the most consistent early sign of this disease process
- Pain around the belly button
- Low-grade fever
- Nausea

Late appendicitis

- Severe pain that has localized to the right, lower portion of the abdomen. Note this is the patient's right side. If the appendix ruptures, the pain can progress to include the entire abdomen.
- High fever
- Severe nausea and vomiting

Patients who are suspected of suffering from appendicitis should be immediately evacuated to the nearest hospital with surgical capabilities. It is much better to be mistaken in this diagnosis than to delay and have the patient suffer severe complications.

After the pain moves to the right, lower quadrant of the abdomen, the pain can be excruciating. Light tapping or bumps in the road in a transport vehicle can be extremely painful for the patient.

If the diagnosis is suspected and help is a day or more away, oral antibiotics such as Ciprofloxacin, along with Metronidazole, may be administered.

Children suffer from this condition at a higher incidence than any other age group. This means that a higher index of suspicion must be maintained in this younger population.

MISCELLANEOUS INFECTIONS

Basically, any infection that may afflict an individual in an urban setting may also do so in a rural one. The only difference remains the lack of diagnostic and treatment resources in a wilderness environment. Below we discuss the more common infections, their diagnosis, and treatment.

EAR INFECTIONS

Three separate chambers exist in the human auditory system, but only the outer two are typically susceptible to infections. Ear infections are divided into two basic categories depending on their location. Infections of the innermost cavity are almost always of viral origin and represent a debilitating condition consisting of loss of balance and spatial awareness along with incapacitating nausea. These patients will have to be transported to the nearest hospital. No effective field treatment exists for this type of infection.

External Ear Infections (Otitis Externa)

Infections of the ear canal external to the eardrum may or may not be caused by bacterial pathogens. In the field, it is virtually impossible to determine if a bacterium is involved unless a fair amount of pus is leaking from the ear opening.

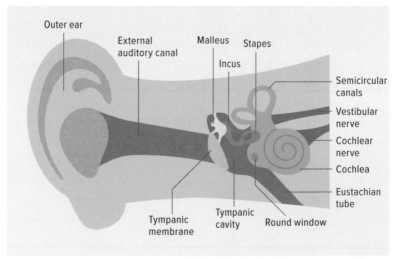

A simplified look at the anatomy of the ear

Signs and Symptoms of Otitis Externa

- Pain in ear canal
- Redness (erythema) inside the ear canal
- Pus oozing from ear canal
- Fever

The field treatment consists of keeping water out of the ear canal and administering acetaminophen and ibuprofen. Antibiotic ear drops are indicated for moderate to severe cases, but they are often unavailable when one is in the backcountry.

Middle Ear Infections (Otitis Media)

Infections of the middle chamber of the auditory complex are typically the result of bacterial or viral pathogens and are potentially more serious than otitis externa. As seen in the image on the facing page, the middle ear is connected to the mouth cavity by way of the Eustachian tubes. This connection allows us to "clear our ears" by yawning or chewing gum with changes in altitude or atmospheric pressure.

The downside of this connection is that the middle ear may become infected by bacteria and/or viruses that travel upwards through the Eustachian tube. Middle ear infections frequently accompany or follow infections of the throat or nasal passages.

Signs and Symptoms of Otitis Media

- Pain in the ear
- Fever
- Hearing difficulty
- Discharge from the ear (indicates the eardrum has ruptured)

Treatment of otitis media consists of oral antibiotics. The initial recommended antibiotic is Augmentin (amoxicillin plus clavulanic acid), 875 mg twice per day for adults who are not allergic to penicillin and amoxicillin, 80 mg for children who are not allergic to penicillin. If these antibiotics

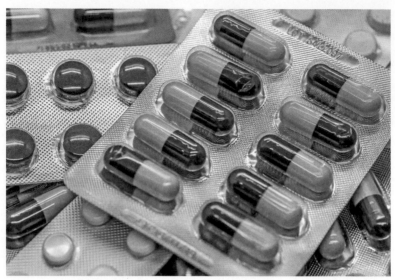
Augmentin is one of the frontline options for a middle ear infection.

are available in the field and evacuation will be delayed, they may be started prior to evaluation by a clinician. These infections usually require a course of 5–14 days depending on the severity of the infection.

URINARY TRACT INFECTIONS

Due to its warm, wet environment, the urinary system represents a prime breeding ground for bacteria. This is especially true for females due to the short length of the tube that carries urine from the bladder to the external environment (urethra). Although males do suffer from urinary tract infections (UTIs) from time to time, the ratio of female-to-male infections is roughly 10:1. Bacteria are essentially always the causative organisms. Specifically, bacteria that inhabit the colon and rectum cause these infections most of the time. Therefore, careful hygiene is required after urination or defecation. More explicitly, females should always wipe front-to-back and clean the genital area daily with soap and water. Males should follow a similar regimen even though their risk for acquiring UTIs is not as great. Treatment of established UTIs in the backcountry can be problematic, while prevention is easy. If a UTI has occurred, the diagnosis is usually straightforward.

Signs and Symptoms of a UTI

- Pain with urination

- Cloudy and/or foul-smelling urine

- Lower abdominal cramping

- Lower back pain (kidney area)

- Frequent urination

- Feeling the need to urinate even when bladder is empty

- Bloody urine

- Fever

As with any disease process, not all signs or symptoms need to be present to make the diagnosis. Treatment should be started as soon as the suspicion is present to prevent the infection from ascending into the kidneys (pyclonephritis). If this occurs, the resultant infection may be very serious and even life-threatening. In an urban setting, the diagnostic and treatment algorithm would include giving a sample to the lab for identification of the specific causative bacteria, followed by starting a broad-spectrum antibiotic. When the bacteria are identified a day or two later, the antibiotic may then be changed to make sure it covers the identified bacterial culprit. Obviously, these tests are not available in the wilderness. For this reason, a specific antibiotic that covers most UTIs may be carried in the first aid kit. The specific antibiotic that kills most bacteria that cause community-acquired UTIs is called trimethoprim/sulfamethoxazole (TMP/SMX {Bactrim, Spectra}). The dose is 160 mg/800 mg twice per day. The usual recommended course of treatment is 7 days. This means that at least 14 pills must be carried to treat a single UTI. The patient should also be encouraged to stay hydrated. Over hydration with copious amounts of water is never recommended due to the risk of electrolyte imbalance. If the urine is relatively clear and the patient is urinating several times per day, that is sufficient.

Patients who do not respond to treatment within several days must seek treatment to analyze the urine and receive appropriate therapy.

SOFT TISSUE INFECTIONS

Essentially any part of the body exposed to the environment is susceptible to becoming infected due to skin and soft tissue injuries or other breaches of the body's defenses. It would require many volumes to detail every possible body location and pathogen that may occur in the backcountry, so we will cover the topic broadly and readers may extrapolate the diagnosis and treatment algorithms to include all body locations.

Cuts, scrapes, and severe bruises may all become secondarily infected, especially in the backcountry where adequate hygiene may be problematic. In general, if an infection coalesces under the skin to form a pocket of pus, the term applied to this is **abscess.** If, however, there is no defined pocket of pus (purulence is the medical term), and a spreading subcutaneous infection occurs instead, the condition is called **cellulitis.**

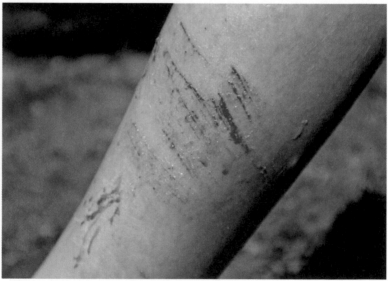
Even minor scrapes can get infected, so cleaning wounds is essential.

Abscesses

If a collection of pus forms in the wilderness setting, the typical best course of action would be to seek care in an emergency department as soon as possible so that it may be opened with a scalpel and drained. If this is not feasible and the infection is worsening, the skin overlying the pus collection may have to be cut open with a scalpel so that the pus may drain.

Although surgical drainage of abscesses is generally best left to doctors, this can be done in the backcountry using a sharp knife if your return to civilization is delayed. This is only recommended if the abscess is not near any major blood vessels and is very superficial. First, gently clean the area (formal sterilization is not required because there is already a pool of pus under the skin), then make a very small cut with the point of a sharp knife to allow the pus to escape. Once this has occurred, use gentle pressure on the sides of the abscess to express the remaining infected liquid. Then apply a clean dressing. Seek definitive medical care immediately.

Cellulitis

Cellulitis, on the other hand, typically responds to appropriate antibiotic administration. As with essentially all other infectious processes encountered in the field, it is not possible to identify the specific causative bacteria. So-called broad-spectrum antibiotics are recommended. This term refers to antibiotics that historically kill the majority of bacteria that commonly cause the particular condition. In the case of cellulitis, several cheap, commonly encountered antibiotics are reasonable first-line choices. For patients not allergic to penicillin, take amoxicillin 250–500 mg three times per day, or cephalexin 500 mg four times per day. For patients allergic to penicillin, take azithromycin 500 mg the first day, then 250 mg. The course of therapy depends on the severity of the infection, but it is generally 5–14 days. Definitive care should be sought for infections that do not show improvement within 2–3 days of starting antibiotics.

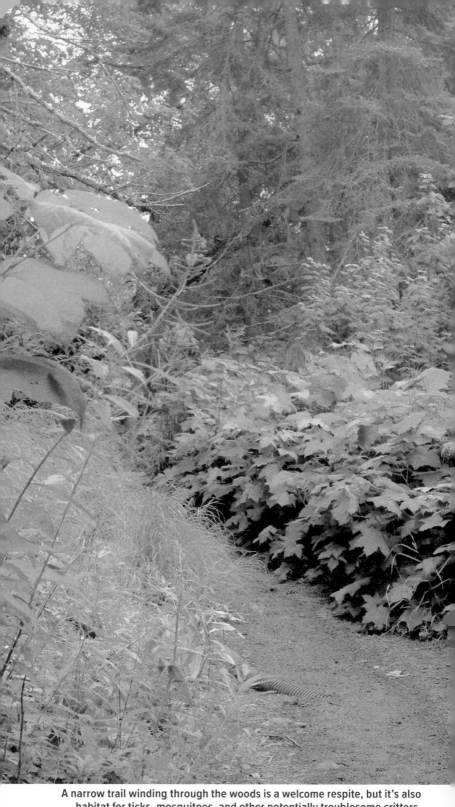

A narrow trail winding through the woods is a welcome respite, but it's also habitat for ticks, mosquitoes, and other potentially troublesome critters.

Ticks, mosquitoes, and other insects are the intermediate hosts for a variety of pathogens that may infect humans. Intermediate hosts means that the animal (insects in this case) carry the virus, bacteria, etc., but do not become ill as a result. They are capable, however, of passing the pathogen on to the definitive host (humans in this case), who do become ill because of the pathogen.

It should be emphasized that insects all over the world carry disease-causing pathogens that may infect humans through bites or stings. Fortunately, the number and severity of diseases transmitted in this matter are relatively small in the United States, but readers are encouraged to educate themselves on the diseases that are prevalent in any country or region they anticipate traveling to. Countries that lie along the equator typically harbor the greatest variety of disease-carrying insects. The farther one travels from the equator, the fewer and generally less severe the infectious possibilities. We will consider only those parasites endemic to the United States in this text.

MOSQUITO-BORNE DISEASES

We have already considered the specific disease processes of encephalitis caused by viruses transmitted by mosquitoes (page 75). Other diseases caused by mosquito-transmitted pathogens include malaria, chikungunya, dengue, yellow fever, West Nile virus, and Zika virus.

With the exception of West Nile virus, the remaining diseases on the list not only rarely occur in the United States, but they are also limited to the hotter, more humid Southern states such as Florida, Alabama, and Georgia. Sporadic outbreaks, especially of malaria, do occur every few years, but the other diseases on the list are mostly seen in travelers returning from tropical climates. West Nile virus remains a persistent problem throughout much of the US.

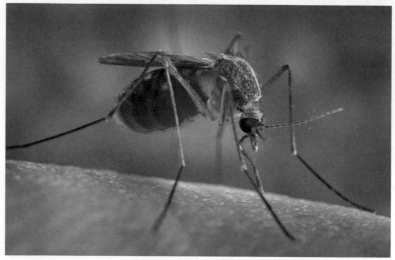
A female *Culex* mosquito, a carrier of the West Nile virus

WEST NILE VIRUS

Signs and Symptoms of West Nile Virus

- Fever
- Skin rash
- Headache
- Severe fatigue
- Muscle/joint aches

Signs and Symptoms of Severe Cases (usually over 50 years of age, immunocompromised)

- Muscle weakness
- Sensory loss in certain body parts
- Paralysis
- Seizures
- Coma/Death

These signs and symptoms are obviously very generic and may, in fact, be the same for several other disease processes. Consider the history of recent mosquito bites along with the appearance of signs and symptoms after the appropriate incubation period (3–14 days). Any patient who displays several of these signs or symptoms should be transported to a care facility familiar with the diagnosis and treatment of this condition. Field treatment consists of rapid evaluation, high index of suspicion for the disease, oral fluids, ibuprofen, and acetaminophen.

The symptomatology for the other mosquito-borne diseases on the list are largely the same as for West Nile virus infections. The field treatment remains the same, and again, rapid transport to a hospital is indicated.

TICK-BORNE DISEASES

As opposed to mosquitoes, ticks generally transmit disease by way of a different pathologic vector. This class of diseases is called rickettsial diseases. Rickettsiae are very small bacteria that can only survive and reproduce inside the cells of a living host. All other bacteria may live independently within the host organism but outside of the cells of that organism. They may even thrive after the host dies, while rickettsiae die shortly after the host does. Just as with mosquitoes, the rickettsiae are transmitted to humans through the bite of a tick infected with the bacteria. A number of closely related tick-borne diseases are listed on the next page. Note that mites may also transmit some

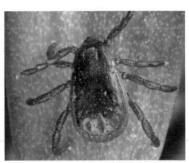

A dog tick, which can be a vector for diseases like Rocky Mountain spotted fever

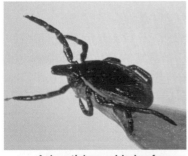

A deer tick on a blade of grass; careful observers may find ticks in a similar posture on vegetation.

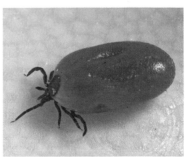

An engorged deer tick adult after a blood meal; the vector for Lyme disease, among others

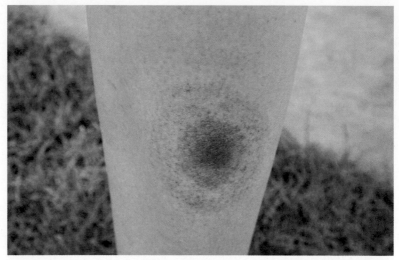

The infamous bull's-eye rash sometimes, but not always, seen in Lyme disease cases

of these diseases, although this is less common in the United States. As with other disease vectors, many other varieties of rickettsial disease occur in other parts of the world, so the world traveler would be well advised to study the endemic diseases of planned travel destinations.

Tick-borne Bacterial Diseases

- Lyme disease
- Rocky Mountain spotted fever (also other named spotted fevers)
- Anaplasmosis
- Ehrlichiosis
- Typhus

Other tick-transmitted diseases do exist in the US, but they are rarer and present in a very similar fashion to the ones mentioned on the list. The exact nomenclature does not matter nearly as much as the prompt recognition that a potentially severe disease process is occurring in the patient. These diseases can be quite serious and even fatal if left untreated. The signs and symptoms of this constellation of diseases is broad, so a high index of suspicion is required in the field. The more common signs and symptoms are listed below.

Classic Triad of Symptoms

- Fever
- Headache
- Rash

Other Possible Symptoms

- Joint/muscle aches
- Neck stiffness/pain
- Nausea/vomiting
- Muscle weakness/paralysis

These bacterial diseases may be treated with antibiotics. These antibiotics must be started as soon as possible, as these infections carry a high mortality rate if left untreated. Rocky Mountain spotted fever, for instance, carries an approximately 30% mortality rate if not treated with appropriate antibiotics.

If one of the aforementioned diseases is suspected, the patient must be transferred immediately to a care facility where the appropriate diagnostic tests and antibiotic therapy can be promptly initiated. As we can see, the signs and symptoms with this group of diseases overlap those of other infectious diseases. It can be very confusing, even

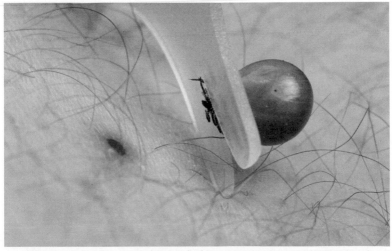

With a tweezers or a pair of hemostats, grasp the tick near its head and pull directly up, removing the head along with the body.

for experienced clinicians to distinguish between various disease processes in the backcountry. The resources are simply not available in a wilderness setting to make an accurate diagnosis.

Fortunately, the antibiotic protocols for tick-borne diseases are mostly the same. Therefore, persons traveling to remote locations for extended periods of time are encouraged to take antibiotics that will cover this group of microorganisms. The antibiotic of choice for those not allergic to it is doxycycline 100 mg twice per day. The recommended course of treatment is 7–14 days depending on the severity of the infection. Doxycycline does cause moderate to extreme cutaneous photosensitivity (skin damage when exposed to direct sunlight). Patients must cover up or stay out of the sun while taking this medication. Definitive medical care should also be sought as soon as possible to confirm the diagnosis and ensure the proper antibiotic regimen is being delivered.

ENVENOMATIONS

Either for personal defense, hunting, or to protect their community, many animals have evolved to possess toxic chemicals in specialized compartments along with efficient delivery systems. Stingers or fangs represent the most common delivery mechanisms. In this section, we will consider the more common venomous animals and some of the field treatment options for those unfortunate enough to have been bitten or stung.

SNAKEBITES

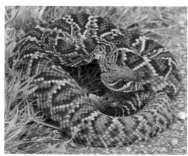

An Eastern Diamondback Rattlesnake
(*Crotalus adamanteus*)

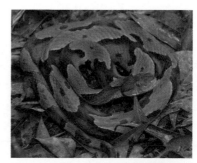

A Copperhead
(*Agkistrodon contortrix*)

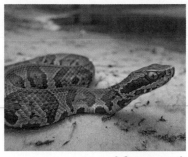

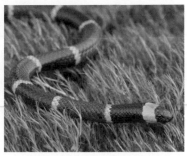

A Cottonmouth
(*Agkistrodon piscivorus*)

A Coral Snake (*Micrurus fulvius*);
remember "red on yellow kills a fellow."

Venomous snakes inhabit most portions of the United States, but the highest concentrations of these animals live in the southern half of the country. All of these animals use fangs to deliver a lethal dose of poison to their small prey. When threatened, this same venom delivery system may be used to ward off a potential attacker. Humans, therefore, are usually bitten by mistake as they inadvertently encroach upon the snake's perceived safety zone. So, unless a human is actively disturbing or threatening the animal by picking it up or attacking it, most bites occur on the lower extremities.

If an individual is traveling in an area known to have a high concentration of venomous snakes, high leather boots, thick long pants, and a walking stick or trekking poles are recommended.

Below is a list of venomous snakes found in the US.

- Rattlesnakes (many varieties)
- Copperheads
- Water moccasins (cottonmouths)
- Coral snakes

Copperheads and water moccasins are generally found in the southeastern part of the US, coral snakes in the southwest, and rattlesnakes are endemic to the entire southern half of the country.

Regardless of the variety of snake, the results are roughly the same. The venomous snakes in the US all deploy proteolytic venoms, which means that the toxin destroys tissue near the bite. Some venoms in other parts of the world are called neurotoxins, which tend to be much more deadly.

The specific identification of each venomous snake in the US is beyond the scope of this text.

Peterson Field Guide to Reptiles and Amphibians of Eastern and Central North America and *Peterson Field Guide to Western Reptiles & Amphibians* are good resources.

Signs and Symptoms of Snake Envenomations

- Extreme pain and swelling around the fang puncture site
- Sweating and increased thirst
- Fever
- Light-headedness
- Racing and/or irregular heart rhythm
- Numbness and/or tingling in the hands and feet
- Seizures
- Decreased level of consciousness
- Coma
- Death

Treatment

Field management of serpent envenomations involves an immediate call for help with transport to the nearest medical facility. The algorithm for rendering aid is outlined below.

- Take a photo of the snake if possible. The definitive treatment for envenomations includes an antivenom that is specific for each species of snake. If unable to take a photo, try to visualize the animal so it can be described to hospital personnel.

- If the bite occurs on an extremity, remove rings, watches, ankle bracelets, etc., on the affected limb. The limb will swell rapidly and massively. If constricting objects are not removed before this occurs, they will be impossible to remove after the swelling ensues. These constricting objects may act as a tourniquet, which can jeopardize the limb and even the patient's life.

- Place a clean dressing over the bite, but do not wrap tape or anything else in a circumferential fashion around the extremity.

- Seek treatment immediately. Do not wait for symptoms to appear.

Actions to Avoid

Some "treatments" that have been handed down over time actually represent maneuvers that may harm the patient. Some of these historical remedies are listed below.

- Do not cut the skin over the wound and/or attempt to suck out the poison. The venom has already been injected deep into the tissues and is irretrievable by any means.

- Do not place a tourniquet or any constricting material around an extremity.

- Do not drink alcohol.

- Do not take any of the NSAIDs (ibuprofen, aspirin, naproxen, Celebrex, etc.). These drugs may exacerbate bleeding tendencies from the poison.

As stated above, the body part that has received the bite will swell. Bleeding may occur in the tissues as well. Except for small children, the elderly, and people with underlying medical conditions, death is unusual from snakebites received in North America. This is distinctly different from bites in other parts of the world, such as southeast Asia and Australia. In such places death can occur, even in robust adults, in less than 30 minutes.

SPIDER BITES

In the United States, only two species of spiders exist that possess the ability to envenomate humans. These are the black widow and the brown recluse. Several other scary-looking spiders, such as the tarantula and the wolf spider, may bite humans, but the bite does not inject toxic substances into the victim.

While black widows may be found throughout the continental US, brown recluses are principally located east of the

Mississippi River. Both species are shy and only bite humans when they come into direct contact with the victim's skin. This is most often the result of the person inadvertently threatening the animal by actions such as putting on clothes that the spider is inhabiting.

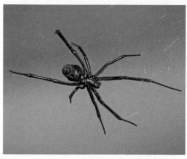

A Black Widow Spider
(likely *Latrodectus hesperus*)

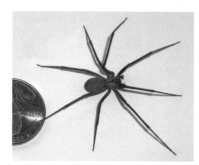

A Brown Recluse (*Loxosceles reclusa*)

Although each spider carries its own distinct venom, they both result in similar symptoms of pain, swelling, and tissue damage surrounding the bite. While neither of the two is typically capable of inflicting a lethal envenomation, both may cause extreme pain and inflammation that can last several weeks. Brown recluse bites, especially, may produce enough tissue damage to require surgery later.

It bears noting that many spider bites are attributed to brown recluses when this is actually not the case. These bites are relatively uncommon, and identifying the offending arachnid is impossible unless you bring the spider in to the emergency department for entomological categorization.

Field treatment consists of identifying the spider with a photo, if possible, and providing transport to the nearest medical facility. Rescuers should follow the Dos and Don'ts mentioned above for snake envenomations. Especially important is to not cut the skin and/or attempt to suck out the poison. Again, this does not work and will only complicate the situation. Also, don't use tourniquets, and be sure to remove any rings or other constricting items if an extremity is involved.

ANAPHYLAXIS

This section deals with the very specific and dangerous situation in which an individual is exposed to a substance that triggers an extreme defensive response by the body to combat this ostensibly harmful substance. In the vast majority of individuals, the substances that cause these extreme reactions are completely benign and do not elicit any sort of system-wide response. Examples include peanuts, wasp or bee stings, cinnamon, and a large variety of less-common substances.

The reaction that such people experience results from an exaggerated release of a certain inflammatory chemical. The exact reason for this unwarranted response is unknown. The medical condition is called anaphylaxis or anaphylactic

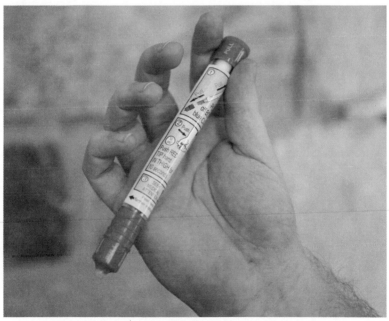

For those with serious allergic reactions, carrying an EpiPen is essential.

shock. The symptoms typically appear seconds after an exposure, such as a bee sting or the ingestion of peanut products. The chemical released from the body's own cells causes hives (raised red bumps on the skin); wheezing, shortness of breath, and use of accessory muscles (neck, intercostal muscles) to breathe; a drop in blood pressure; and, if left untreated, respiratory collapse and death.

Death can occur within only a few minutes of the onset of symptoms, so treatment must be initiated immediately. Fortunately, most people know if they are prone to anaphylactic episodes. These events are so severe that people have already experienced the cycle of anaphylaxis and successful treatment at least once. Because of this, these individuals will usually carry their own medication wherever they go.

This medication is called epinephrine and may only be administered by injection into a muscle (called intramuscular injection). This should ideally be done by the patient, if they are able. Failing this, qualified medical personnel should inject the drug. If there is no medically trained person available, a bystander may be forced to do it in order to save the person's life.

Giving such an injection is not difficult, but as with any other medical intervention, there are risks associated with it. Obviously, these risks are insignificant when compared to someone's life, but several caveats should be kept in mind.

- The injection should only be directly into exposed skin, never through clothing.

- The safest injection site is the outside (lateral) aspect of the shoulder.

- The next safest option is the outside (lateral) portion of the thigh.

- Don't worry about cleaning the skin before giving the injection. This is a life-saving maneuver.

- Pop the needle through the skin quickly, then inject the contents of the syringe into the muscle.

- A drop or two of blood may appear at the injection site— it is of no consequence.

Hopefully the patient's symptoms will begin to subside within 2–3 minutes. If oxygen is available, it should be administered as long as the patient experiences any respiratory distress.

One critically important factor to keep in mind: If the injection of epinephrine does "cure" the patient, the rescuer should be watchful for the return of potentially life-threatening symptoms. This does happen occasionally. The reason is that some agents (antigens) that precipitate an anaphylactic crisis can linger in the body for quite some time. Epinephrine, on the other hand, has an extremely short duration of action within the body (called the half-life).

Therefore, the "curative" chemical (epinephrine) may disappear from the bloodstream before the inciting agent (antigen) does, thus allowing for a return of symptoms. If this happens, a second dose of epinephrine may be administered.

It cannot be overemphasized how important it is to accurately diagnose an anaphylactic reaction before giving an EpiPen injection. Epinephrine can be a potentially life-threatening drug if given to the wrong individual in the wrong circumstance. If a rescuer does suspect that such a reaction is occurring, they should call for trained medical personnel as they initiate treatment.

ANIMAL BITES AND RABIES

Essentially all wild creatures possess the ability to cause us harm through the biting process. With the exception of primates, animals use their mouth for almost all purposes that relate to investigating food sources, acquiring food, attacking threats, and defending territory. They are typically much faster and frequently much stronger than we are. In short, they are best left alone.

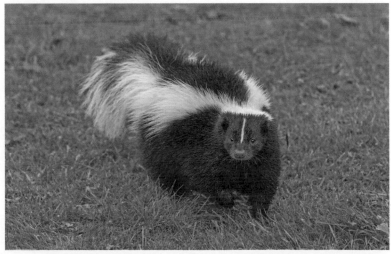

Skunks, raccoons, foxes, and bats are the most common rabies carriers.

Aside from the physical consequences of a bite, such as bleeding and tissue damage, animal bites may transmit diseases. The bacteria in the mouth of the creature can initiate a local infectious process, but the saliva of an animal may also carry a more insidious and dangerous pathogen: The **rabies virus.**

Rabies is the name of the disease caused by a particular virus that is contained within the saliva of infected animals. The virus is in the family of Rhabdoviruses and attacks the central nervous system of infected animals, including humans. Other similar viruses may be transmitted this way, but in the US rabies is far and away the predominant viral vector.

Many animals may carry the disease, but skunks, bats, and foxes are frequent carriers. Animals that progress to the end stage of the disease become disoriented and are frequently aggressive. All animals that exhibit unusual behavior, such as lack of fear of humans, aggression, etc., should be assumed to be infected with the rabies virus.

If an individual has been bitten or scratched by a wild animal, first aid should be administered in the form of stopping the bleeding by direct pressure, washing and bandaging the wound, and seeking medical attention immediately.

All individuals who have been bitten or scratched in this manner must be assumed to have contracted the disease. Treatment must begin immediately and consists of a series of painful injections administered over a period of two weeks.

The reason for this haste is that, left untreated, rabies is essentially 100% fatal. There is no known cure once symptoms have begun.

Worldwide, trauma represents the number one killer of people less than 45 years of age and is the fourth-leading cause of premature death across the entire population. In the backcountry, the percentage of trauma deaths and injuries are even greater. For this reason, it is critical that a potential rescuer possess a solid framework of decision-making when approaching a trauma scene. Obviously, no text or even occasional multiday training can prepare a nonmedical person for every traumatic eventuality. The goal here is to provide the reader with a basic framework from which to develop an efficient, timely algorithm when confronted with a critically injured patient.

What we are aiming for are rescuers who can reproduce the same rapid assessment for each injured person they are tasked to assist, followed by (or concurrent with) quick, effective treatment, while arranging for additional resources as needed. This sounds prohibitively complicated, but the foundation for every scenario is the same. Well-executed rescue efforts use this foundation as a springboard to develop a coherent treatment and evacuation plan for whatever eventuality ensues.

Trying to assist an individual who has just sustained a significant traumatic event should elicit an extreme stress response in any compassionate person. To mitigate this, it is recommended to follow some simple mental pathways. The sequences are described here.

Trauma is divided into two basic categories: **Penetrating** versus **Blunt.** Penetrating injuries include gunshot wounds, impalements, stabbings, arrow injuries, etc. Blunt injuries include everything else, including falls, motor vehicle accidents, blast injuries, etc. There are several miscellaneous categories, such as **burns** and **lightning strikes,** that will also be covered in this text.

As a whole, penetrating injuries tend to be either rapidly fatal or not immediately life-threatening. Blunt injuries, on the other hand, are often more complex, subtle, and difficult to diagnose. The internal damage caused by blunt trauma also may not manifest immediately, and the patient may deteriorate after some time, even though the person may appear to be rock-stable. Exceptions may occur when it comes to both of these generalizations.

PENETRATING TRAUMA

With penetrating trauma, there is always an entrance wound and sometimes an exit wound. The structures and organs in harm's way become much more apparent with these types of injuries. We further divide penetrating wounds into high velocity versus low velocity. High-velocity injuries are caused by bullets in the majority of cases. Why is this distinction important? Low-velocity injuries, such as those caused by knives or arrows, only damage tissue that is directly in the path of the invading object. It becomes relatively easy to assess potential injury patterns in this case. Only a millimeter or two of tissue adjacent to the foreign object will be compromised in such cases.

Gunshot wounds, however, represent a completely different situation. Due to their extremely high rate of travel, bullets cause an extensive amount of tissue destruction outside the actual path of the projectile. This damage extends in a cylindrical geometry around the bullet's path. This cylinder of destruction is called *cavitation* in trauma surgery circles. The degree of tissue destruction is related to the muzzle velocity of the firearm. At first blush, it would seem that the size of the bullet would determine the potential for injury or death. Although this does play a role, it is a relatively minor one.

The kinetic energy of the bullet is what determines the volume of tissue destroyed in the individual who has been shot.

The equation that governs this phenomenon is **KE = 1/2 MV2,** or in layman's terms, kinetic energy equals half of the mass of the object times velocity squared.

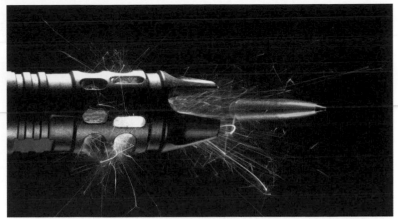

AR-15 bullet leaving a rifle

As we can see, while increasing the mass of a bullet will cause a proportionate increase in destructive energy transmitted, increasing the velocity will increase the energy transfer exponentially. Here is an example:

A 9mm handgun bullet weighs approximately 8 grams and has a muzzle velocity of 1,000 ft/sec.

An AR-15 assault rifle uses a .223 (muzzle diameter in inches) bullet, which weighs around 4 grams. The muzzle velocity of this weapon is about 3,000 ft/sec.

Using the formula above (we won't trouble with units, just comparing the proportionate energy transfer), we see that the 9mm handgun with the large bullet delivers 4M energy units. The AR-15 with a bullet that weighs half of that of the 9mm round delivers 18M energy units. The tiny AR-15 bullet will destroy 4½ times the tissue of the larger 9mm one!

Why do we bother with the physics of this? As a practical matter, due to the great disparity in tissue destruction, it is unusual for an individual to survive a body-mass gunshot wound with a high-velocity weapon. Torso wounds caused by handguns or lower-velocity rounds convey a much higher survival opportunity.

Treatment of these and other penetrating injuries will be covered in subsequent chapters.

LOW-VELOCITY AND IMPALEMENT INJURIES

Unlike high-velocity injuries, objects traveling at lower speeds (including arrows) only damage the tissue directly in the path of the projectile. Therefore, unless the object severs a major artery or penetrates a major organ, the victim will quite likely survive with timely intervention.

One critical bit of counsel on impalement injuries or other penetrating wounds where the object remains in the victim's body cannot be overstated: *Never* remove a penetrating foreign body in the field. The reason for this is as follows: impaling objects may invade a body part in a non-lethal location but may partially injure a major blood vessel or vital organ. The object, while in place within the body, may serve as a buttress to prevent major blood loss. If this object is removed, it may uncover the hole in the blood vessel or major organ with subsequent death due to hemorrhage. In medical terms, this foreign object while left in situ (in place) serves to tamponade the potential hemorrhage.

In the field, there is no way to predict whether an impaling object is indeed preventing a major artery or vein from bleeding; therefore, such objects should only be removed in the operating room by a trauma surgeon.

BLUNT TRAUMA

Falls from height and falling objects represent most blunt traumatic injuries that one may encounter in the backcountry. The increased use of OHVs (Off-Highway Vehicles) has added a component of high-velocity impact and roll-over injury patterns to the mix. In contrast to penetrating

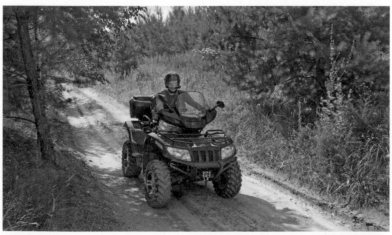

As OHV use has risen, so have accidents.

injuries, blunt trauma represents a more difficult assessment situation for the backcountry responder. Because of these potential diagnostic conundrums, it is helpful to remember some basic diagnostic algorithms to help focus us during periods of stress and to efficiently allow us to assess, treat, and evacuate blunt trauma victims in the backcountry.

The first thing to consider after confirming that the patient has suffered a blunt versus penetrating injury is whether or not the injury is isolated to one body part or involves multiple areas on the body—called multisystem involvement.

We will consider isolated injuries to occur only to the extremities, as head/neck/torso injuries frequently involve multiple organ systems. Isolated injuries include such things as fractures, dislocations, burns, crush injuries, and lacerations. These will all be discussed later in this chapter.

Multisystem injuries carry an increased potential for life-threatening consequences and should alert the rescuer to a heightened need for rapid assessment and transfer to a tertiary care facility. Specific injuries to all organ systems will be addressed in this chapter, but the initial assessment of all patients with potentially severe and/or multisystem injuries *always* starts with the ABCs. One of the most important reasons to emphasize this point involves what are called *distracting injuries.*

DISTRACTING INJURIES

When a victim has suffered multiple injuries, it is natural for rescuers rendering aid to have their attention drawn to the most obvious or painful injury. This frequently leads to more subtle but potentially more serious injuries being missed.

Therefore, as rescuers, we start with ABC (Airway, Breathing, Circulation) assessments as described on pages 1–8. When those entities are addressed appropriately, we begin a rapid head-to-toe evaluation of the patient. It is during this phase of the process that we examine and treat injuries other than those encountered during the ABC assessment (primary survey). Any distracting injuries, such as angulated extremity fractures, will be managed during this phase. This top-to-bottom examination is called the secondary survey (see sidebar, page 117). Several points are worth mentioning here. First, the

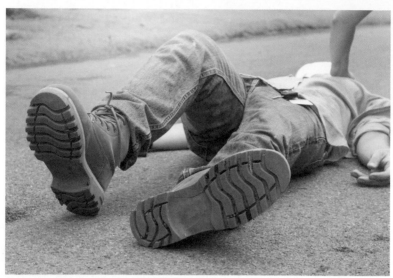
When faced with an emergency, follow the steps shown on the facing page.

survey should ideally be completed before starting treatment to not forget to completely examine the patient. This survey should take no more than 60 seconds or so to avoid delay in treatment. The second caveat is to examine underneath clothes as well as the patient's dorsal surfaces (back of head, neck, torso, buttocks, and legs). Many serious injuries have been missed because rescuers were either too embarrassed to look at the skin surfaces underneath clothes or did not take the time to log roll a patient to look for occult injuries.

At this point, if the patient is as stable as possible given the resources at hand, they should be interrogated very briefly regarding medical history. Should the patient's level of consciousness not allow for this, any person with the patient who has knowledge of their medical condition should be questioned. If cell service exists, call a family member who might possess that information.

Although a detailed history is always beneficial to obtain at some point, for the purposes of field treatment and for relaying salient data to additional responders or hospital personnel, three questions will suffice initially:

1) Does the patient have any ongoing illnesses or medical conditions such as heart disease, diabetes, hypertension, cancer, pulmonary disease, etc.?

2) Does the patient take any medications and have those medications been taken appropriately today?

3) Is the patient allergic to medication or allergens found in the environment?

These questions will provide adequate information to all concerned without wasting time either at the scene or during a radio relay.

WHEN FACED WITH A POTENTIAL MEDICAL EMERGENCY, FOLLOW THESE STEPS:

First, conduct a primary survey: Airway, Breathing, Circulation (see pages 1–8).

Then, perform a secondary survey:

1) Start with a head-to-toe exam, including dorsal surfaces and underneath clothes.

2) Compile a brief medical history of conditions (high blood pressure, diabetes, heart disease, etc.).

3) Create a list of any medications the patient takes regularly, and ask if they have been taken as directed today.

4) Note any allergies to medications or environmental triggers.

A plethora of acronyms exists as mnemonic for the sequence above, but again, multiple acronyms tend to blend together and it becomes difficult to remember which acronym belongs with each circumstance. Therefore, starting with the ABCs and then continuing with the sequence above seems to not represent an overly burdensome memory exercise. Notecards in a backpack or in the notes app of a smartphone can be useful as well.

FIELD REPORT

A rescue team is called for a climber who has fallen near the summit of one of the 14ers in southwest Colorado. His fall is reported as a tumbling 50-foot fall onto a scree field. Initial assessment from the hasty team dispatched to assess the individual reveals only a "tib-fib" fracture of the lower portion of the right leg. The patient is in extreme pain and the team appropriately splints the injured extremity. Additional personnel and equipment arrive within 20 minutes of the arrival of the first team. A thorough ABC and secondary assessment by this second team reveal crepitus, or air trapped in the subcutaneous space indicating a pneumothorax (collapsed lung), and bruising over the chest wall just below and to the side of the collarbone, with mild pain on palpation. The patient states he does not feel much pain here because his leg hurts so badly. He denies breathing problems. The patient is immediately placed on oxygen by nasal cannula, the receiving hospital and ambulance crew are notified, and the patient is rapidly transported by wheeled litter to the waiting EMS crew.

The lesson here is that patients may not even be aware of a life-threatening injury due to a less-significant distracting injury that commandeers the attention of both the victim and the first responders. These types of situations are exactly why the ABCs must be performed before assessing and treating individual injuries, even if those injuries are extremely painful and gross.

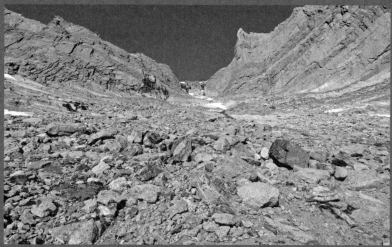

Unforgiving terrain in the Colorado Rockies

HEAD, FACIAL, AND SPINAL CORD TRAUMA

Brain and spinal cord injuries represent a major portion of the trauma-related morbidity and mortality worldwide. One reason for this is that, even though the central nervous system (brain and attached spinal cord) is protected on all sides by a bony endoskeleton (skull and vertebral column), it has an extremely limited capacity to heal or regenerate, unlike other structures. This means that whatever deficit occurs after an injury to these structures is likely to persist permanently. Some mitigating treatments can be administered in trauma centers, but the caveat here is that the patient must receive definitive care in a hospital dedicated to central nervous system injuries as quickly as possible.

The salient aspects of field treatment include rapid assessment and rapid evacuation. Specific injuries are discussed below.

HEAD INJURIES

We can think of the brain as the central processing unit of our bodies. All received information in terms of environmental stimuli is processed here, and then motor signals are distributed to the appropriate organ system. A grain of sand touches our cornea and we blink. We spot a rock falling toward us and we dodge out of the way. It is for these basic survival instincts, as well as the ability for higher thought processes, that it is imperative that the very fragile brain be protected. This is where the skull comes into play. The average skull thickness in adults ranges 6–8 mm. While this bony structure does provide some protection against minor traumas, it is startling how little force is required to cause permanent neurologic injury. We will again divide injury patterns into blunt versus penetrating.

Blunt Force Head Injuries

As the brain is a very soft and fragile organ contained within the skull, it is extremely susceptible to bruising because of trauma to the skull. Any blow with force sufficient to cause bruising or laceration to the scalp may, in turn, cause damage to the brain. Not only is the brain matter immediately beneath the trauma at risk, but so is the brain as it sloshes against the opposite wall of the skull. This injury represents a so-called *contrecoup* injury.

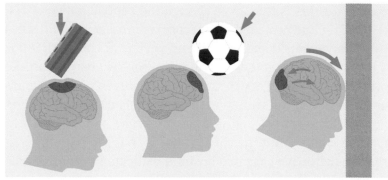

A few examples of how a contrecoup injury can occur

These injuries may occur in any portion of the brain, including the cerebellum and brainstem, which controls our most basic functions, including respiration and cardiac activity. Such injuries may merely cause bruising of the brain matter, but they can also initiate massive bleeding, leading to stroke and death. Any number of other symptoms may also occur, from no symptoms to headaches, nausea, loss of motor function or sensation, and blindness.

How do we know when to seek treatment for someone who has sustained a blow to the head? Below are basic guidelines for transferring a patient for in-hospital care:

- Loss of consciousness

- Any of the above-referenced symptoms that occur after blunt head trauma, especially nausea, progressive headache, or loss of any motor function

- Any mechanism that is worrisome due to significant trauma that may not be immediately apparent. An example would be someone who has fallen more than 10 feet and landed on their head, but was not knocked unconscious and who does not manifest any symptoms.

- Anyone who has sustained significant trauma to the temporal area, whether or not symptoms are manifested. Several high-profile celebrities have died after sustaining injuries to the temporal area but not complaining of any problems.

Unfortunately, patients in the latter two categories often have life-threatening injuries overlooked by hospital personnel exactly because they don't display any symptoms. Such injuries frequently manifest many hours later, after the patient has gone home. All such patients warrant a head CT scan and overnight observation in a hospital with neurosurgical services available.

An additional, very useful field as well as in-hospital diagnostic schematic is called the **Glasgow Coma Score (GCS).** This table represents a quick and accurate way to determine the initial severity of a head injury. To arrive at a score, and thus a degree of severity, the rescuer evaluates three separate components of the patient's motor and sensory functioning. They include Best Eye Response, Best Motor Response, and Best Verbal Response. The table on page 122 clarifies this.

To achieve the correct number, the rescuer should observe the victim's response to verbal commands (Open your eyes!, Squeeze my hand!). It is acceptable to pinch the patient's fingernail to elicit a pain response if they are unconscious.

Adding the best response from each of the three columns gives a number from 3–15. The severity of the head injury can then be accurately reported using this number. The grading is as follows:

Mild: 13–15   **Moderate:** 9–12   **Severe:** 8 and below

Patients with severe head injuries must be considered for the insertion of a definitive airway (intubation, cricothyroidotomy) by an advanced trained individual. Obviously, the urgency of transport is partially dependent on the Glasgow Coma Score.

Field Treatment

Three basic maneuvers exist for field treatment of blunt head trauma:

- Elevate head above the level of the heart. This helps mitigate any swelling that may be occurring inside the skull.

- Provide oxygen, either by nasal cannula or face mask. Especially for patients who sustain head injuries at high altitude, supplemental oxygen may help stabilize the situation until definitive care can be reached.

- Rapid transport. It is difficult to overstate the importance of this. Again, even asymptomatic patients who have sustained significant head trauma may deteriorate without warning. This can lead to death in a matter of minutes.

Eye Response

Scale	Score
Eyes open spontaneously	4
Eyes open to verbal command or speech	3
Eyes open to pain	2
No eye opening	1

Verbal Response

Scale	Score
Orientated	5
Confused conversation but able to answer questions	4
Inappropriate responses	3
Incomprehensible sound or speech	2
No verbal response	1

Motor Response

Scale	Score
Obeys commands for movements	6
Purposeful movement to painful stimulus	5
Withdraws from pain	4
Abnormal flexion or decorticate posture	3
Extensor response or decerebrate posture	2
No motor response	1

FIELD REPORT

The mountain rescue team is called out for a 72-year-old man who has received a blow to the head from a rock that a member of his party accidentally dislodged above him. He has suffered a 2–3-minute loss of consciousness. The team arrives 45 minutes later to find the patient alert and joking with family members. He does complain of dizziness and is unsteady on his feet. Due to these complaints, the patient is placed in a wheeled litter and taken down the very difficult and steep terrain toward the trail. The rescue vehicle lies some 20 minutes beyond.

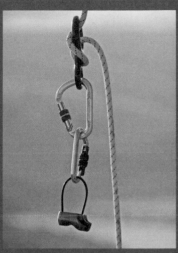

Suddenly, the patient's level of consciousness descends into a comatose state. He is not responsive to verbal or painful stimuli. Some seconds later, he begins to vomit. Oxygen was previously placed, and he is turned on his side to prevent aspiration and allow personnel to clear his airway.

Climbing is a beloved pastime, but it can prove dangerous.

Within a minute, the patient has agonal respirations (gasping for air). These ineffective attempts to breathe cease quickly thereafter. All resuscitation efforts fail, and the patient is pronounced deceased after a prolonged period of Advanced Cardiac Life Support (ACLS) maneuvers.

The takeaway from this actual occurrence is that all significant traumatic events to the brain and/or spinal cord should be treated as life-threatening emergencies. This often does not turn out to be the case, but there is absolutely no way to determine this in the field. The most expeditious method of evacuation must be employed in such circumstances.

Penetrating Head Injuries

Any part of the body, including the skull, can be impaled by a foreign object. The rule regarding not removing an impaling object becomes even more critical in this setting. Patients frequently survive even devastating cranial impalements as long as the object is removed in the operating room by neurosurgeons—and nowhere else.

FACIAL INJURIES

In anatomical terms, not only does the face serve as the interface between the brain and the outside world to receive visual, olfactory (smell), and taste stimuli, but it also serves as a sort of bumper to protect the brain from injury due to frontal trauma. The bones in the face can absorb a surprising amount of force before the brain suffers damage. Any bone in the face may break, but there exists a subset of these that can result in potentially life-threatening airway compromise. Collectively, these are referred to as Le Fort fractures.

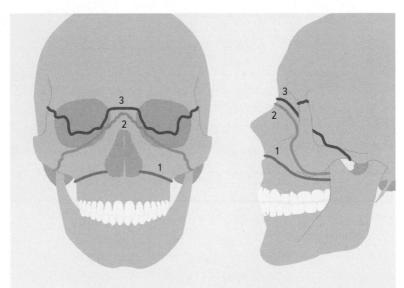

Three types of Le Fort fractures

These are fractures of the mid-face that result in collapse of the central portion of the face. This structural instability may obstruct the patient's airway, necessitating action from rescuers to allow for more normal breathing. As we see in the image on page 124, the three varieties of fracture increase in complexity along with the increasing number. It is not important to memorize or even understand the fracture pattern; the only thing a rescuer needs to do is to examine the face carefully and to prevent the unstable anatomy from interfering with the patient's breathing. If the rescuer notices obvious fractures of the face and the patient appears to be having trouble breathing, either due to blood running down the throat or the face pressing inwards into the mouth, it is vital to turn the patient onto their side, clear the mouth with a sideways sweeping motion, and to manually pull the "free-floating" facial fragments outward. This will obviously be an extremely unsettling experience for the person performing this maneuver, but it can be lifesaving.

Eye Injuries

Major eye injuries occur with either a blow to the eye socket or an object that becomes impaled in the globe. Because the eyeball rests in a bony cup, a frontal force may actually rupture the eye itself. The eyeball is filled with a viscous liquid and an ocular rupture may manifest after significant trauma, resulting in excruciating pain, bleeding from the eye, as well as extrusion of this viscous (vitreous) liquid.

Field treatment of such injuries includes completely covering the affected eye along with the other eye. This is important because the eyes are incapable of independent movement; therefore, if the unaffected eye looks in a certain direction, both eyes will track in the same direction. This will cause significantly more pain in the affected eye and may injure it further. Immediate transfer to a trauma center is paramount for such injuries.

Penetrating or impalement injuries to the eye are treated in much the same way as blunt injuries. Covering both

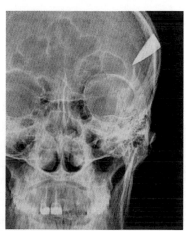

A CT Scan image of an impalement injury near the eye

eyes and immediate transfer to a tertiary care facility are the only tools at the rescuer's disposal here. For objects that become impaled in the eye, it is again critical that rescuers do not attempt to remove the object. This can have disastrous results in terms of hemorrhage and preserving the patient's eyesight. What should be done in these cases is to construct a stabilizing bandage with tape and something like a paper cup. If very long, the penetrating object should be gently secured with tape to the cup or similar protective device, which, in turn, should be securely taped to the patient's face. Again, it is very important to cover the patient's other eye so that no further damage to the injured eye occurs.

Any of the many other facial bones may be broken, but the only field treatment consists of hemorrhage control by direct pressure, bandage if appropriate, and transfer to the appropriate medical facility.

SPINAL CORD INJURIES

Injuries to the spinal cord represent a devastating situation for the patient. The spinal cord is protected 360 degrees by the vertebral bones, along with a series of layered, thick muscles. Therefore, any injury to the spinal cord can only occur after a tremendous amount of force has been absorbed by the body. Once the spinal cord itself has been injured, it is extremely difficult, if not impossible, for it to heal itself.

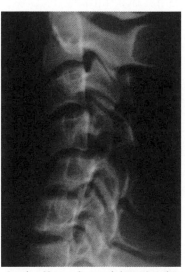

A spine X-ray after an injury showing cervical subluxation

Damage to the spinal cord may occur after one part of the torso is violently moved while the remaining body is held stationary, with severe crush injuries, or by penetrating injuries.

With any sort of blunt-force trauma, the cord itself could be bruised or completely severed. Although patients may improve significantly with only bruising of the cord, transections of the cord result in permanent motor and sensory loss below the level of the injury. In the field, it is impossible to distinguish between these two situations, and the treatment remains the same. The treatment for penetrating or impaling injuries to the vertebral column, including the spinal cord, are the same for such injuries in other parts of the body: hemorrhage control, stabilization of the impaling object, and rapid transport.

Signs and Symptoms of Spinal Cord Injury

- Appropriate history (i.e., severe trauma, penetrating object)
- Pain at the transection site
- No motor function below the level of the injury
- No sensation below the level of the injury
- Paradoxical low heart rate and low blood pressure

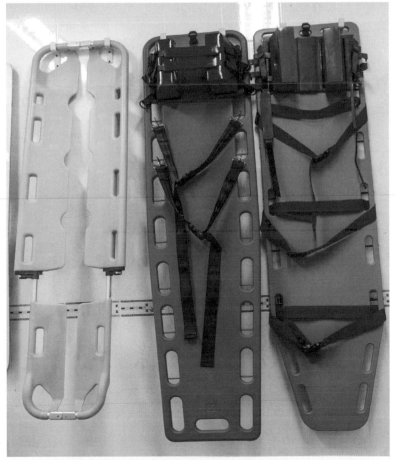

Various spinal boards for stabilization of potential spinal cord injuries

Any injury to the spinal cord requires urgent stabilization of the entire vertebral column, along with the most rapid transport possible to a level 1 trauma center with neurosurgical capabilities. Any decompression of the spinal cord or other surgical maneuvers must be performed within a few hours of injury to have any hope of minimizing the post-injury morbidity.

Patients may be initially transported on firm backboards (with appropriate padding), but longer transports should be accomplished with the patient on a firm but not rock-hard litter to prevent pressure-related injuries. A good option that most search-and-rescue teams have, for instance, would be a vacuum mat (bean bag) pad, which conforms to the contour of the patent. The air is sucked out of the mat after it has been molded to the patient. After all air has been removed, the mat stays in the shape it was molded into until the air valve is opened, allowing air to reenter. These mats are great for stabilizing not only spinal columns, but also extremity injuries.

THORACIC TRAUMA

We can think of the thoracic cavity as a more-or-less cylindrical cage that serves the dual purpose of protecting the heart, lungs, and other vital organs contained therein, along with expanding and contracting with each breath to allow the process of respiration to occur. The boundaries of this cage include the paired diaphragm muscles that separate the thoracic cavity from the abdominal cavity, the spinal column and rib cage, and finally the neck.

As with any other body part, the thoracic region is susceptible to both blunt and penetrating trauma.

BLUNT THORACIC INJURIES

Due to the proportionally large size of the thoracic space, it is a common site to receive blunt-force trauma because of falls, falling objects, motor vehicle crashes, and other accidents. Although the bony endoskeleton (ribs, vertebrae, sternum) provides a significant degree of protection for the underlying heart and lungs, there is a limit to its ability to withstand extreme traumatic stress.

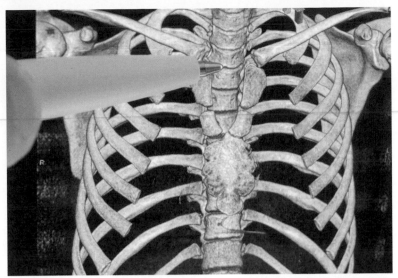
A CT image of the thoracic cavity

An additional factor to consider when evaluating a patient in the backcountry who has sustained some sort of injury to the chest cavity is age. As we age, the muscles that help protect this vital area, such as those between the ribs (intercostal muscles), back muscles (latissimus dorsi, rhomboids, etc.), and side muscles (serratus anterior), atrophy and therefore provide less of an effective buffer. Just as with other bones of the body, the ribs and vertebrae become more brittle with age and tend to break with significantly lower applied stressors, which can lead to bony fragments causing internal harm to the heart or lungs.

A blow to the chest to a fit 25-year-old, for instance, may merely result in some bruising and discomfort. That same blow applied to the chest of an 85-year-old may cause a potentially fatal injury. Specific injury patterns are considered below.

Rib Fractures

Broken ribs represent the most common injury to the thoracic zone. As described above, they occur significantly more frequently in the elderly due to thinning and loss of mineralization of the bones. On the other end of the spectrum, rib fractures in infants are distinctly uncommon due to the surprising elasticity of the bones in this age group.

As a rule, isolated rib fractures do not represent a medical urgency, as, other than pain medications, there is little to be done in the way of treatment. Having said that, more than one rib fracture may cause enough discomfort to limit the patient's respiratory effort, which, in turn, may lead to the development of pneumonia after a few days. In these circumstances, the patient should be transferred to a hospital for consideration of special analgesic injections.

What absolutely should not be done in the field is any sort of circumferential chest wrapping. This will only further constrict the patient's breathing. The patient should be evacuated expeditiously—walking is fine in the absence of other mitigating injuries.

More than two rib fractures bring us into the arena of more significant thoracic crush injuries. The pain involved with multiple rib fractures increases exponentially. This level of pain essentially always results in rapid, shallow, ineffective respirations. Additionally, the force required to fracture multiple ribs frequently results in underlying pulmonary contusion (bruising of the lung), which can progress rapidly to respiratory failure. For these reasons, these injuries usually mandate a helicopter evacuation.

Another factor to consider is that, with an increase in the number of fractured ribs, there exists an increasing chance of a collapsed lung (pneumothorax) due to a broken rib fragment penetrating into the chest cavity and injuring the lung. These injuries will be discussed later in this chapter.

The evaluation and diagnosis of rib fractures are usually straightforward: with the area exposed completely, the affected area can be *gently* palpated. Point or localized tenderness will be diagnostic in this case. Pushing deeper may elicit a sensation of bone scraping on bone, but there is no reason to put a patient through this pain.

Flail Chest

A special situation occurs with massive blunt trauma to the chest in which four or more contiguous ribs are fractured in two or more places. This results in a section of the rib cage losing its connection with the rest of the bony thoracic infrastructure. This disconnected section then moves

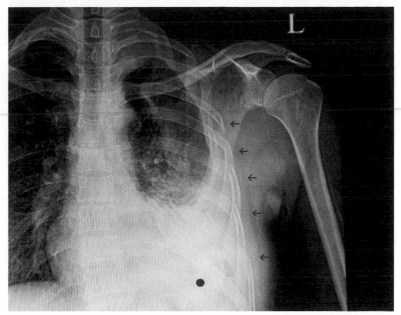

Multiple broken ribs (red arrows) and flail chest on an X-ray

paradoxically during the respiratory cycle. In other words, this damaged portion sucks in when the rest of the rib cage expands outward, and vice versa (see above). This is a true emergency. Not only is it quite likely that these patients have suffered accompanying underlying injuries, but the dysfunctional respiratory mechanics quickly lead to outright breathing failure and death. These patients must be treated by personnel with advanced training and equipment usually within an hour at the most.

Hemothorax and Pneumothorax

Severe damage to the chest cavity may result in one or both sides of the chest filling up with blood or air. Hemothorax is the term when blood is involved, while pneumothorax is used when air is the culprit. A quick treatise on thoracic anatomy will help us better understand these processes, along with how to treat them.

The lungs rest in either side of the thoracic cavity encased in a double-walled membrane called pleura. We can think of it this way: if we take our fist and push it into the center of a very large balloon without popping it, our fist will be covered by two layers of balloon material.

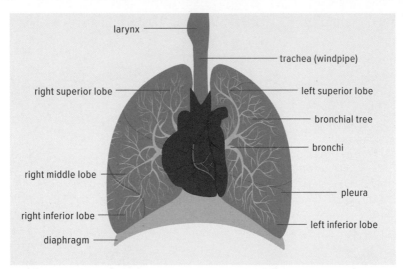

A simplified look at lung anatomy

Metaphorically, the fist represents the lung, and the two plastic layers of the balloon are equivalent to the two pleural membranes. It is the space between the pleural layers that can fill with either blood or air, thus compressing the healthy lung tissue and compromising its ability to expand and contract.

When an object such as a rib fragment is forced inward, it may puncture both pleural membranes as well as the lung itself. If this occurs, air may leak out of the lung under pressure higher than the space between the two pleural membranes and cause an accumulation of air. This accumulation of air is called a pneumothorax. There are three distinct expressions of this condition that we will consider below.

Simple Pneumothorax Fortunately for us, our tissues, including the above-mentioned pleural membranes, possess a remarkable ability to seal small- to medium-size puncture wounds. In the example above, when a fractured rib penetrates the lung, the hole is usually small enough that the injured membrane will close the breach within a few minutes. This results in a small volume of air trapped in the space between the two pleural membranes (pleural space), but the accumulation does not continue due to the incredible self-sealing membrane. What we have then is a partial collapse of the affected lung, but it's usually not enough to cause problems in the field (see image to follow).

The diagnosis of this problem consists of a good history from the patient or bystander, along with our *Look, Listen, Feel* algorithm. Examine the exposed chest cavity for signs of trauma, listen to breathing sounds with a stethoscope (if available) to compare both sides, and gently palpate the entire chest cavity. What you are feeling for here are indications of rib fractures but also, and more importantly, a specific sensation that only occurs with pneumothoraxes. When air leaks out of the lung, it will often seep into the tissues just under the skin. If this area is palpated, it feels exactly like popping Rice Krispies underneath a layer of Saran Wrap. The term for this is *crepitus.* This finding is unmistakable and occurs with no other traumatic event—at least for the purposes of the first responder in the backcountry.

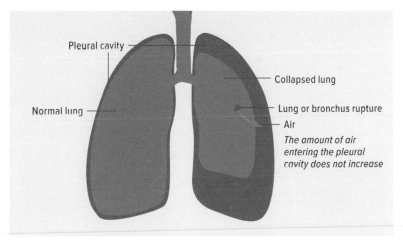

Simple pneumothorax

This finding allows the rescuer to report with certainty that the patient has suffered a traumatic lung collapse. This provides an additional degree of urgency to the evacuation process. Field treatment includes supplemental oxygen and rapid evacuation.

Open Pneumothorax   The second variety of pneumothorax occurs when the lung, along with both pleural membranes, is punctured as described above; however, in this instance, there is an opening in the skin that connects with the inside of the chest cavity. This opening allows the flow of air in both directions—inside out, and outside in.

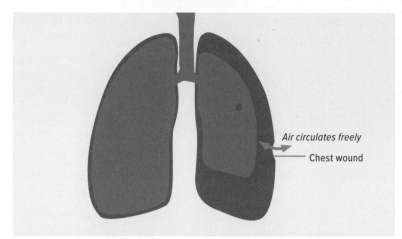

Air circulates freely
Chest wound

Open pneumothorax, also known as a sucking chest wound

This type of wound is sometimes referred to as a sucking chest wound. Even in the medical community, there's an almost frantic need to cover such a wound. It can be admittedly disconcerting not only to see such a wound, but to hear air moving in and out of the chest cavity. Indeed, it is appropriate to cover the opening with an occlusive (airtight) dressing. This can be accomplished in the field by cutting a piece of a waterproof raincoat, water bladder, or other similarly airtight material to fit over the wound, and then taping it in place.

One vital caveat exists here. It is critical that the rescuer note the character and rate of the patient's respirations before AND after placing such a dressing. It is a mixed bag whether an airtight dressing helps or hurts in such a situation. For example, if leakage of air continues from the lung itself, and the rescuer occludes the only point of relief of the pressure that builds up within the chest cavity by placing an occlusive dressing, then that air will accumulate until the patient dies. This is called a tension pneumothorax (covered below).

Therefore, after the dressing is placed, the patient should be questioned as to exactly how their respirations compare to before the bandage was applied, and the rescuer should count the number of respirations per minute and compare that to the number before the dressing was applied.

If the patient's respiratory condition deteriorates after the dressing is in place, it should be immediately removed. Although an open chest wound is disturbing to onlookers, it can be definitively treated in a hospital setting.

Tension Pneumothorax   Continuing with increasing severity of the various types of pneumothoraxes, we come to the most serious of all: the tension pneumothorax. As described above, this situation occurs when a traumatic event has punctured the lung and at least the pleural membrane immediately adjacent to the lung (visceral pleura), but the chest wall is intact. This situation is very similar to when an empty balloon is attached to a helium cylinder, the valve of the tank is opened, and the balloon fills. In the situation of the tension pneumothorax, the chest cavity (pleural space) represents the balloon. It fills with air, but unlike the balloon on the tank, the chest cavity has a very limited capacity to expand, and the high-pressure air compresses the lung on the affected side until death occurs.

This situation can be lethal in a very short time, often less than 30 minutes. It must be recognized and definitively dealt with immediately if the patient's life is to be saved. The only treatment for this is to decompress the chest cavity with a large-caliber tube inserted through the chest wall (tube thoracostomy). This procedure is beyond the scope of the wilderness first responder, but rescuers on the scene may at least recognize the problem and call for immediate resources to address the problem.

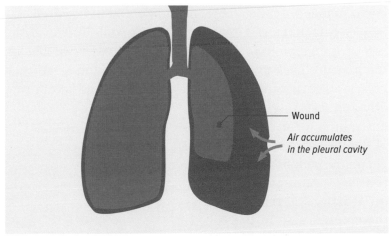

Wound

Air accumulates in the pleural cavity

Tension pneumothorax

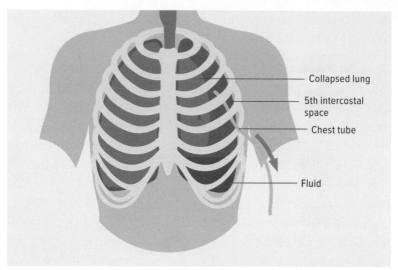

A simplified graphic of a tube thoracostomy

Each rib has its own medium-size artery that runs along its undersurface. External forces that fracture ribs frequently disrupt these so-called intercostal arteries, which then bleed into the chest cavity. If enough blood accumulates in this space, the lung may be compressed to the point of impairing respiration. This is called a hemothorax. It can be exceedingly difficult to differentiate a hemothorax from a pneumothorax in the field. Once again, the patient should be examined with the *Look, Listen, Feel* algorithm. If either a hemothorax or pneumothorax is suspected, a special diagnostic maneuver called *finger percussion* should be used.

For this diagnostic technique, the middle finger of the rescuer's nondominant hand is placed between two ribs on the patient's back away from the vertebrae and large back muscles. The middle finger of the dominant hand is very rapidly and forcefully thumped down directly on the middle of the three bones of the finger on the patient's chest.

This technique should immediately be repeated on the opposite side in the corresponding position. The tone of the sound should be compared. If one has not

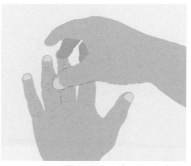

The percussion technique

performed this procedure before, it can be difficult to distinguish tonal differences, but the basics are this: for a normal, uninjured person, a finger percussion should elicit a mid-range, hollow sound. Since blood (or any liquid) muffles sound waves, percussion in the setting of a hemothorax will produce a dull thud when compared to the other side. A pneumothorax, on the other hand, elicits a very distinctive, higher-pitched reverberation, similar to the sound of a mid-range drum. This particular sound is called tympany.

Individuals should practice this technique on a partner so as not to try and sort out the different sounds on a critically injured patient in the backcountry for the first time.

There is little rescuers can do to treat a hemothorax in the field. Again, the takeaway is to diagnose the injury as accurately as possible so that advanced personnel may have an idea of what they are dealing with. Supplemental oxygen, positioning the patient in a mild head-up position, and emergent evacuation represent the cornerstones of field treatment for this condition.

PENETRATING THORACIC INJURIES

The treatment algorithms for penetrating trauma to the chest cavity are much the same as for blunt injuries. The caveat to remember here is to **never** remove an impaling object in the field. The object may be staunching a bleeding vessel within the chest cavity, or even preventing a simple pneumothorax from becoming a tension pneumothorax. Any long object penetrating the thoracic cavity may be carefully cut to a length that will allow for easier transport, or, if this is not possible, the responding team must devise a way to transport the patient along with the impaling object in place. It may appear as though the patient has no chance for survival with such an injury, but there have been several instances where patients have survived seemingly lethal impalements. Such injuries obviously require an efficient, expeditious, and well-coordinated field response.

The rescuers should ensure that no further damage is done by the offending object by having one rescuer dedicated to stabilizing the object manually. Supplemental oxygen and air evacuation are paramount in this setting.

FIELD REPORT

As I was finishing up my surgical residency, our team received, without warning, an individual who had been impaled by a 6-inch diameter fence post. This piece of wood entered his body just at the lower-left rib cage area and exited through the back. Roughly 2 feet of the post protruded from each side of his body. After quickly preparing him for surgery, we rushed him into the operating room where we carefully but rapidly opened his thoracic and abdominal cavities; stopped the bleeding; removed the post along with his spleen, a portion of his stomach, and intestines; and repaired massive holes in his diaphragm muscle and lung. He walked out of the hospital two weeks later.

ABDOMINAL AND PELVIC TRAUMA

As we continue downward on the body, we will next consider injuries to the abdominal and pelvic areas. The abdominal cavity houses a variety of disparate organ systems, all of which are at risk in the event of a concentrated, forceful blow to the front, sides, and even the back.

The contents of the abdomen are protected in the back by the vertebral column, the broad back muscles, and a bit by the ribs. The walls of the flanks and the front are composed of heavy cross-layered muscles that provide an effective shield against low-energy traumatic insults. As with all human tissue, when the protective ability of these barriers is breached by an extreme force, internal damage ensues. Falls from heights, rockfall, motor vehicle accidents, and other high-energy transfer incidents may result in internal abdominal injuries. The salient issue with all intra-abdominal traumatic injuries is that they are essentially all serious and potentially life-threatening. The two main categories of damage to abdominal organs include hemorrhage and rupture of the gastrointestinal tract.

INTRA-ABDOMINAL HEMORRHAGE

Bleeding that occurs within the confines of the abdominal cavity originates from either rupture of the spleen, liver, or kidneys (strictly speaking, the kidneys are separated from the abdominal cavity by a membrane, but we will include them

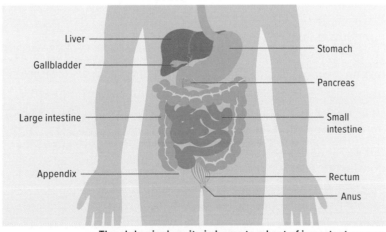

The abdominal cavity is home to a host of important organs.

here) or from disruption of a major artery or vein contained therein. Anatomically, the liver resides on the patient's right side, just under the diaphragm; the spleen occupies a similar position on the patient's left side; and the paired kidneys are in the mid–low back region. Therefore, any significant blow to these areas should elicit a high index of suspicion for injury to these organs.

How do you know if one or more of these organs is damaged and bleeding? They are located very deep in the abdominal cavity and are therefore not able to be felt directly. The answer lies in a careful reconstruction of the traumatic event, either by questioning the patient or bystander, along with a very careful exam. The patient's skin should be exposed to the extent that a visual inspection may be performed. Take care to only expose the skin long enough for an exam if hypothermia is a concern. The entire abdomen, including the flanks, should be visually inspected. You are looking for any indications of trauma, including bruising, abrasions, and lacerations.

Next, *gently* palpate (push on) the entire surface of the abdomen. This should be done carefully and systematically. We typically divide the front surface of the abdominal cavity into quadrants: right upper, left upper, right lower, and left lower. If the rescuer is kneeling

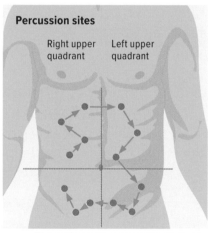

Percussion sites

Right upper quadrant   Left upper quadrant

The main quadrants of the abdomen

on the patient's right side, it is usually ergonomically natural to start with the left upper quadrant and work sequentially in a clockwise fashion. It doesn't matter how it's done, as long as it's accomplished in a logical, thorough manner. If the patient is conscious, he or she can indicate any areas of discomfort or outright pain.

There are some very specific signs that intra-abdominal hemorrhage has occurred or is ongoing. First, your initial survey should have included a set of vital signs, including heart rate. A very fast heart rate (greater than 100 bpm in adults) is a strong indicator of significant blood loss. External signs of trauma on the skin of the abdomen, coupled with pain elicited by palpation, are also representative of a deeper injury. Finally, two specific signs, if present, indicate massive bleeding within the abdominal cavity. This bleeding generally originates from the spleen or liver, as these two organs contain a disproportionately large volume of blood.

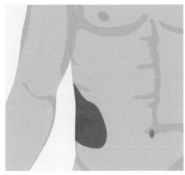

Grey Turner's sign

The first of these signs is called **Grey Turner's sign.** When a large volume of blood accumulates inside the abdomen, this blood pools along the sides in some naturally occurring "gutters" by the colon. After an hour or so, this blood may be visible as bruising along the flanks.

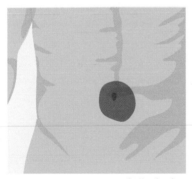

Cullen's sign

The second sign, which often accompanies Grey Turner's sign, is called **Cullen's sign.** In this instance, the accumulated blood travels along vascular pathways and congregates around the belly button.

Of note with both of these signs is that the area where the blood accumulates is remote from the injury area. In other words, these areas will typically not be painful when palpated because the injury (again usually to the liver or spleen) occurs at a distance from these outward signs.

Hemorrhage significant enough to produce these two signs usually also causes abdominal distention.

These signs indicate a degree of bleeding that warrants immediate transport via helicopter if available.

Field treatment involves rapid identification, supplemental oxygen, and immediate evacuation. No other maneuvers will be beneficial in the backcountry.

Many other possible sites of bleeding exist within the abdominal cavity. It is quite difficult to differentiate between such sources in the backcountry, but the clinical signs and symptoms are similar: abdominal distention and pain, rapid pulse, and a drop in blood pressure if the bleeding is significant enough.

PELVIC TRAUMA

The pelvis is a roughly circular matrix of bones to which are attached the large bones of the legs as well as the vertebral column that forms the support structure for the upper half of the body.

Due to this central location, the pelvis represents an incredibly strong structure. However, any force great enough to disrupt the integrity of this structure imparts a potentially

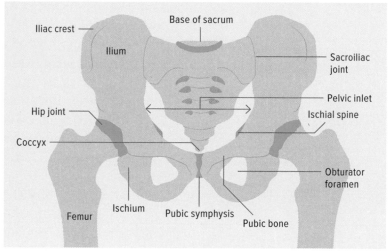

A simplified look at the anatomy of the pelvis

lethal force. An additional point to remember is that, because of its continuous nature, any break in the ring will produce at least two discrete fracture sites. Think of it this way: if you take a circular, 10-inch diameter piece of hard pasta and compress it from two sides, the ring will not just break in one location, but in multiple ones. Therefore, except for a glancing blow that merely shears off a chunk of bone, any direct force from the front, back, or side that breaks this bony ring will do so in more than one spot.

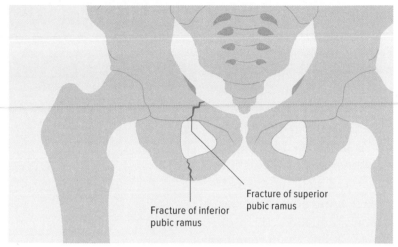

Fracture of superior pubic ramus

Fracture of inferior pubic ramus

Common fractures of the pelvic bones

The most immediately lethal variant of pelvic fracture is called an open book fracture. This fracture occurs when an extreme force has been applied to the pelvis in a front-to-back orientation. Car crashes, pinnings from rockfall, and other accidents are the sorts of forces required to produce this sort of calamity. Anatomically, what we see is a complete disruption of the cartilage in the very front of the pelvis—the pubic symphysis. The corresponding fracture(s) are in the back of the pelvis, usually at the sacroiliac joints.

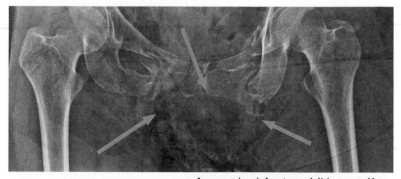

An open book fracture visible on an X-ray

Such a fracture typically tears some of the large veins contained within the sacrum. This results in massive hemorrhage in this area, which can be rapidly fatal if not treated expeditiously.

Diagnosis of significant pelvic fractures, such as an open book fracture, includes a history of appropriate trauma combined with a specific diagnostic maneuver called a *pelvic rock* test. This test is performed by the rescuer kneeling at the victim's waist and placing the palm of each hand on either side of the pelvis on top of the prominent bony outcroppings located just above the groin on each side. The anatomic

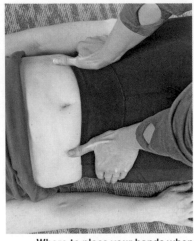

Where to place your hands when conducting a pelvic rock test

term for these prominences is the Anterior Superior Iliac Crests (ASIC). The rescuer then compresses downward with both hands gently but firmly. As the pelvic ring is normally completely inflexible, any movement of flexion of the pelvic ring, especially in the front, indicates a fracture.

Additional Indications of a Severe Pelvic Fracture

- Pain in the pelvic region around a suspected fracture
- Distention and possibly bluish discoloration of the lower abdomen between the belly button and pubis
- Blood at the urinary outlet orifice (called the urethral meatus)
- Vital signs indicating massive hemorrhage (i.e., increased heart rate and declining blood pressure)

Treatment of suspected pelvic fractures includes very rapid diagnosis followed by circumferential compression of the pelvic region. This maneuver is called *pelvic binding.* It is difficult to overemphasize the rapidity of treatment needed in order to maximize the patient's survival chances. Bleeding of this magnitude may result in a nonrecoverable deterioration in a matter of minutes.

Hospitals and rescue organizations typically are supplied with specialized pelvic binders for these fractures.

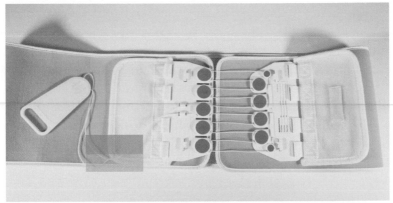

A pelvic binder

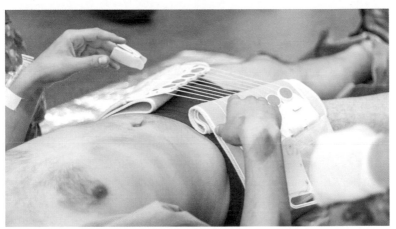

Placement of a pelvic binder; note the low placement location.

As we can see, the binder is placed directly over the pubic symphysis and below the level of the ASICs mentioned above. The usual mistake is for the binder to be positioned too high. Placement should be verified by more than one rescuer, if possible. The binder should be tightened essentially as much as possible. The goal of the binder is to compress the pelvis and thus minimize the space available within the pelvic interior. This will, in turn, limit the available volume of dead space for blood to accumulate. It won't be possible to prevent a large amount of blood from accumulating—the goal is to hopefully stem the flow enough for the patient to make it alive to the hospital where definitive treatment may be accomplished. This sort of process is known as tamponading a bleeding source and is applicable to other bleeding sites as well.

Obviously in the backcountry, such specialized equipment is rarely available. Therefore, rapid improvisation is in order. This is one situation where thoughtfulness about this potential situation would be helpful before embarking on a backcountry adventure so that a frantic search for an appropriate pelvic binder does not overly delay immediate treatment.

While a binder is being fashioned, it would be appropriate for a strong rescuer or two to manually compress the pelvis from side-to-side.

Any fairly broad material, such as the waist belt of a backpack or an ensolite pad cut to about 4–6 inches wide, will suffice. Webbing or rope is then cinched tightly over this wider material. This wide padding serves to mitigate tissue damage that a thin material such as a rope may cause. A rescuer may stand on each side of the patient with the rope or whatever beneath the patient and crossing at the pelvis. The rope is pulled tight, then the rescuers walk in the same direction around the patient to set the tension. This may be done several times to provide enough friction so that the tension is maintained until the rope may be secured.

A backpack may even be used, at least initially, by placing the waist belt directly over the symphysis and tightening it as much as possible. Most modern backpacks have plastic buckles that are too flimsy to provide enough compression, but if this is all that is available, it may be worth a try—at least until a sturdier substitute is fashioned. Again, the key here is compressing the pelvis as quickly and firmly as possible. If the first iteration of your improvised setup does not appear to be adequate, leave it in place while you construct a better one.

Any binder configuration will only temporize the bleeding from such a severe pelvic fracture. The patient must be immediately transferred to a trauma center for lifesaving definitive care.

FIELD REPORT

A call comes in for a level 1 trauma. A pedestrian has been hit by a car traveling at approximately 35 miles per hour. She manifests a waxing and waning level of consciousness and has obvious trauma to the left side of her thorax and multiple deformities of the entire left arm. She has a suspected pelvic fracture. Field treatment consists of oxygen, a pelvic binder, and rapid transport.

In the trauma bay at the emergency department, she moans incoherently; airway is intact, breathing is rapid and shallow, and there's no obvious external bleeding source. Her Glasgow Coma Score is 12 (see section on head trauma, page 122); blood pressure is 110/70; pulse is 96.

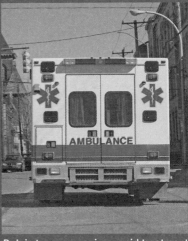

Pelvic trauma requires rapid treatment and professional care.

Oxygen by face mask is administered. Physical exam and X-ray indicate multiple rib fractures on the left and a large pneumothorax. A tube is quickly placed between the ribs into the thoracic cavity to decompress the collapsed lung. The pelvic binder is loosened so that a rapid examination of the pelvis may be performed. An open book pelvic fracture is encountered. Within seconds of loosening the binder, the pulse increases to 130 bpm and the blood pressure drops to 90/60. The binder is firmly reapplied with rapid hemodynamic improvement.

The patient is transferred to a level 1 trauma center where she undergoes multiple operations and endures a difficult multiweek stay in the hospital. She eventually survives and recovers, although not to the level of health she enjoyed prior to the accident.

The takeaway is that the ABCs must be evaluated and addressed quickly and in order, and that a firm pelvic binder placed in the field may be lifesaving for severe fractures.

EXTREMITY TRAUMA

As we continue our examination of traumatic conditions from central to more peripheral locations, we finally come to the consideration of injuries to the arms and legs. Note that the anatomy of the arms and hands are remarkably similar to that of the legs and feet. Given this fact, any condition that affects an upper extremity may be treated in a similar fashion to the same condition that occurs in a lower extremity and vice versa. Obvious differences exist in terms of size, weight bearing, and other factors.

BLUNT EXTREMITY TRAUMA

Blunt force injuries to an extremity may produce a broad array of tissue damage from minor scrapes and bruising, all the way to the loss of an extremity and even death. Fortunately, we have evolved in such a way that the most vital structures are protected by the heavy bones that form the internal structural support of the extremities. These vital structures include the large arteries that supply oxygenated, nutrient-rich blood to the tissues of each extremity; the large veins that return oxygen-depleted, toxin-laden blood back to the heart and lungs; and the nerves that supply motor function and sensation to the muscles and soft tissues.

These important structures are tucked medial (closer to the body core) of the large bones so that even high-impact forces may be absorbed by the bones, thus protecting the vital neurovascular tissues. Car bumpers work in a similar way— the outer elements are sacrificed to protect the occupants.

In an evolutionary sense, this configuration has ensured that more humans reach the age of reproduction instead of succumbing to minor injuries during childhood.

For our purposes, it means that more patients stand a chance of surviving to reach a tertiary care facility despite high energy–transfer insults.

An example of this is seen at the top of the next page, which shows the large single brachial artery of the upper extremity protected by the upper arm bone—the humerus. After the brachial artery splits into the two large arteries of the forearm, the radial and ulnar arteries, we see that these two arteries are similarly protected by the corresponding forearm bones called the radius and ulna.

As the arteries continue to split into smaller and smaller arteries, the importance of being protected by a specific bone diminishes. This is because traumatic injury of these small arteries rarely results in a life-threatening hemorrhage.

Although veins carry a corresponding volume of blood as the arteries, only the very large veins are similarly protected. This is due to the very low pressure in the veins. Injuries to even larger-diameter veins will frequently not result in lethal hemorrhage, as clots will seal the defect in the venous wall in the setting of such low pressure. This is why we observe veins just under the skin of lean individuals while the arteries are buried deep inside. The high arterial pressure prevents adequate clot formation when the integrity of these structures is breached.

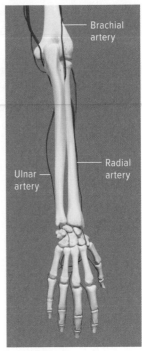

An image of the main arteries in the hands and arm

We will now consider specific extremity injuries.

FRACTURES

Bony fractures involving any location on the body may be broadly categorized as follows:

Simple Fractures Similar to snapping a dry stick, bones may be parted by applying sufficient lateral force to overcome their innate ability to withstand such a force (breaking strength). As with all variations of fractures listed below, such an injury will produce pain, swelling, and discoloration near the fracture site.

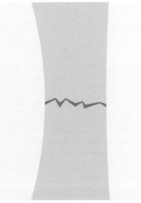

A simple or closed fracture

Open Fractures These sorts of fractures have been referred to in the past as compound fractures. The word *open* is more descriptive and has replaced the more antiquated nomenclature. This situation results when a breach in the skin overlying the fracture occurs. This open wound may be the result of the external force that caused the fracture or be due to one of the bony fragments that has been forced outward with enough energy to open the skin.

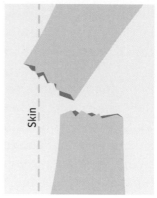

Open fracture

Along with the symptoms of pain, swelling, and discoloration, these wounds pose a much greater risk of infection and must be treated expeditiously to avoid this potential complication. Gently brush away any debris, and/or gently wash the wound with clean water by pouring it over the site. Never attempt to dig into the wound or force water into the deep tissues. This markedly increases the risk of potentially severe soft-tissue infections.

After cleaning the wound, apply a clean, loose dressing and stabilize it, as for simple fractures.

Comminuted Fractures Bones that have sustained severe external force may be pulverized into a large number of fragments. The risk of permanent damage or even loss of the extremity increases with such a fracture due to a compromise of the blood supply and or damage to the nerves. Such a fracture produces a boggy, pulpy feel to the site of injury. Treatment is the same as for either simple or open fractures as appropriate.

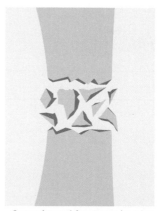

Comminuted fractures involve many bone fragments.

Extremity fractures occur when external forces such as direct blows, torsion, or crushing events exceed the ability of the bones to withstand such forces. Depending on the bone, these forces can range from minimal to quite large. Obviously, the larger the bone, the more force is required to break it and the more serious the consequences for the patient.

General Points Concerning Fractures

First, fracture sites should *never* be wrapped with any compressive bandage directly over the site. Broken bones elicit an extreme swelling response, and any constricting, circumferential wrap may unknowingly block off the blood supply to the extremity beyond the wrap. Nerve damage may also occur.

Elevating the injured extremity above the level of the heart, if possible, will also help reduce swelling. Ice or cold compresses gently laid over the fracture site may also help with the pain and swelling.

It's also very important to verify the neurovascular integrity of the extremity after the injury and especially after the rescuer has finished field treatment. What does this mean? As mentioned previously, large arteries and nerves course close to the large bones to supply blood and to allow for sensation and motor function of the muscles of the arm. If any of these structures are compromised either by the injury itself, or by our treatment, we need to know about it as soon as possible.

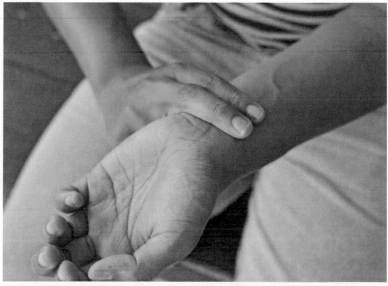

Checking for a pulse on the wrist

To check for adequacy of blood flow past the injury, we can feel for the pulse and/or check for what is called capillary refill. To see if the patient has a pulse, and thus adequate blood flow, gently but firmly feel for the radial pulse at the wrist on the same side as the patient's thumb.

If a pulse is felt, that is all that is required. If the environment is cold, it may be difficult to feel the pulse. Additional personnel may try if any question arises.

Capillary refill may also determine the adequacy of perfusion. To check this, simply compress the pad of any of the patient's fingers, let go quickly, and see if the whiteness caused by the rescuer's compression is quickly replaced by a normal pink color. For darker-skinned individuals, the nail may be compressed in a similar way. This "pinking up" should occur within 2 seconds if blood supply is normal. Again, if the patient is very cold, this may take a bit longer. A trick is to compare whatever maneuver that is performed on the injured side with the noninjured side. Even if the pulse or capillary refill are not ideal, if they are equal to the uninjured extremity, then perfusion may be assumed to be adequate.

To check if the nerves are intact, simply ask the patient to wiggle their fingers, then see if the patient, with eyes closed or looking away, can feel you touching a specific finger without seeing where you are touching it.

If the neurovascular exam described above is normal after the injury, but abnormal after you have applied any stabilization maneuvers, remove the sling and padding, reassess, and construct a different stabilization methodology.

If the patient is not allergic, ibuprofen may be useful to reduce pain and swelling.

Upper Extremity Fractures

Humerus The humerus is the large bone in the upper arm that extends from the shoulder joint to the elbow. Although quite strong, this bone is susceptible to fracture primarily due to direct blows or falls with an outstretched arm.

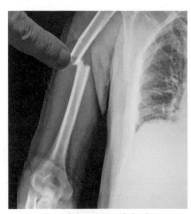
A fracture of the humerus

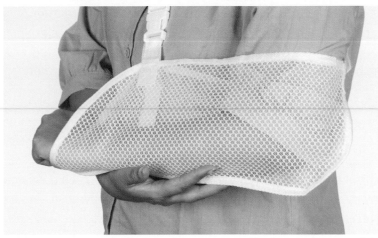

A sling in use with an arm injury

Field diagnosis is relatively straightforward. Appropriate history of trauma, coupled with severe pain and swelling at the fracture site, will give the rescuer all the clues necessary to assume a fracture has occurred and treat it accordingly. The majority of humeral fractures happen in the very middle of the bone—called mid-shaft humerus fractures. If the fracture is severe enough, the upper arm may deviate in an abnormal geometry (angulated fracture).

Field treatment of such an injury includes stabilizing the fracture so that the broken fragments do not move against each other and the surrounding soft tissue and thus create more pain and damage to adjacent structures. The patient can direct the exact positioning to minimize discomfort, but typically a sling fashioned from a piece of clothing, such as a jacket or extra shirt, along with appropriate padding to maintain the elbow joint 1–2 inches away from the patient's side, works the best. The arm in the sling may also be wrapped loosely with an ACE wrap or something similar to stabilize the arm even more. An important point to remember is that, with all fractures, the fracture site, along with the joints proximal and distal to the fracture, must be immobilized. This is because extremity muscles usually cross the joint on either side of a long bone, such as the humerus, in order to provide motion to the distal portion of the extremity. An example would be the biceps muscle of the arm. It runs along the humerus but attaches to the tip of the scapula (shoulder blade) as well as one of the large bones of the forearm (the radius). Thus, the muscle crosses the joint on either side of a humeral fracture. If the rescuer only stabilizes the exact spot where the fracture occurs, muscles such as the bicep can still engage, which would in turn move the broken bones and potentially cause more pain and tissue damage.

Clavicle Fractures   Fractures of the clavicle (collarbone) occur with some regularity due to its very exposed position in the body. The main evolutionary function of this bone is to protect the very large underlying artery and vein—the subclavian vessels. We can think of the function of this protective structure in much the same way as the bumper of a car. The bumper crumples with an impact to minimize the force transmitted to the occupants.

Falling causes the vast majority of these fractures. Skiing, mountain biking, trail running, etc., are some of the more frequent activities associated with this injury.

This fracture is very easy to recognize, as the collarbone will be visually deformed. The typical pain and swelling associated with all fractures occur here as well.

Treatment consists of the usual ice, ibuprofen, and immobility. An arm sling is the preferred method of immobilizing the injured part. Medical care should be immediately sought as well.

Forearm Fractures   The structural support of the forearm is provided by two long, strong bones called the radius and the ulna. The radius is the bone located on the thumb side and the ulna on the pinky side. Although considerable forces are still required to break these bones, they do sustain fractures at a higher rate than the humerus due to their more exposed location and smaller diameter.

Forearm fractures are treated in a corresponding fashion to those involving the humerus or long bones of the lower extremities. The cornerstone of field treatment includes stabilization of the fracture site as well as the joints above and below the injury. In this case, the joints include the elbow and the wrist. The most convenient way to accomplish this is an improvised sling. This has the added benefit of immobilizing the shoulder, which will further reduce the motion of the affected arm. Elevation, ice, and ibuprofen will help.

As stated previously, neurovascular integrity distal to the injury site must be assessed by checking the radial pulse and motor/sensory function of the fingers.

Wrist Fractures   The wrist is composed of eight very small, interlocking bones. These structures allow for an incredible range of movement and flexibility in this very important body part. Several of these bones are prone to breaking, however, even with relatively minor trauma. Field diagnosis is similar to other fracture locations—history of trauma, pain, swelling, and bruising. Ice, elevation, ibuprofen, and sling immobilization are again in order.

Hand and Finger Fractures   As we move farther from the body core, the bones become smaller, more exposed to potential trauma, and more fragile. These conditions allow for a significantly higher number of hand and finger fractures as compared to humerus fractures, for instance. Fortunately, these more distal fractures are not as dangerous to the patient as the more proximal ones.

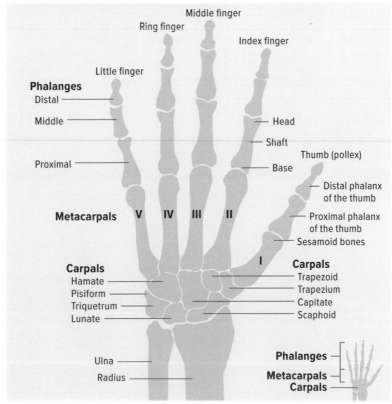

Bones of the wrist and hand

Fractures of the long bones of the hand (metacarpal bones) are common, especially with falls. For example, an outstretched hand may smack against a rock when you're crossing a creek with ice-covered, exposed rocks.

Treatment remains the same as for the other fractures covered earlier. The entire hand, including the fingers, may be immobilized with a piece of closed-cell foam or similar material. Remember to not wrap the area tightly and to reassess the fingertips at frequent intervals to make sure there is adequate blood supply.

Each of the four long fingers contains three separate bones (phalangeal bones). The thumb only has two such bones. This means that 14 small bones on each hand are exposed to potential fracture in what is often a very hostile backcountry environment. No wonder phalangeal (finger) fractures happen with such frequency.

Field treatment follows the same treatment algorithm as for fractures at other locations. In addition, the injured finger(s) may be loosely taped to adjacent, uninjured digits.

Lower Extremity Fractures

Fractures of the leg are treated in a similar fashion to those of the upper extremities. The obvious difference here is that it is very unusual for a patient to be able to walk, so it's more difficult to get help from the backcountry with a lower extremity fracture. The bony anatomy of the leg is very similar to that of the arm. The specific anatomic details are shown in the image on the image below.

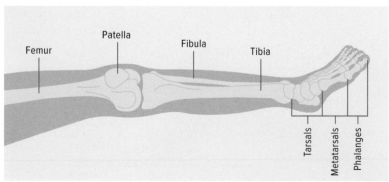

Simplified leg skeletal anatomy

The principles of fracture management are exactly the same for lower extremity fractures as for upper extremity ones. The joints above and below should be stabilized, and the injured part should be gently cleaned if an open wound is present. It bears repeating to not wrap anything tightly around the extremity due to inevitable swelling. The patient will require personnel to transport them out of the back-country either by air or ground transport.

One situation that occurs with more frequency in the lower leg than in the upper leg or any portion of the arm is a condition called compartment syndrome.

Compartment Syndrome

As discussed, fractures elicit massive swelling due to fluid and blood that leak into the surrounding soft tissues. Where there is ample room for expansion, this does not present a problem. The difficulties ensue when that swelling occurs and there is no room for the tissues to expand. This becomes most problematic below the knee for the following reasons: the lower leg is divided into four separate compartments by tough, non-yielding sheets of tissue called fascia. These fascial sheets separate the four compartments, three of which contain one of the three arteries that split off from the main single leg artery. When the tibia is fractured, the swelling may be so intense within one or more of the compartments that the pressure in that compartment exceeds that of the pressure within the artery. When that occurs, the artery becomes blocked and the leg distal to the blockage becomes deprived of blood. This will result in the death of the tissue beyond the blocked artery within minutes to hours. If all three arteries become blocked, the entire lower leg may die very quickly.

This same situation may occur in the upper leg or the arm, but it is much less common.

The diagnosis of this condition is confirmed by verifying a broken lower leg and observing swelling in that area. The tissues all around the lower leg will be extremely tense and disproportionately painful. Compared to the other foot, the injured one will typically feel colder, look paler, and have diminished or absent pulses. The capillary refill, normally less than 2 seconds, will be delayed. To finalize the diagnosis, the patient's foot is gently dorsiflexed (toes pushed toward the face) by a rescuer. Extreme pain in the calf away from the fracture site confirms the field diagnosis.

This situation represents a true surgical emergency. The patient must be transferred to a trauma center within 2–3 hours to save the leg, and even the patient's life. Emergency surgery will need to be performed to relieve the pressure and allow blood to flow again.

Besides emergency evacuation, ice and elevation will help mitigate the swelling.

FIELD REPORT

A world-class athlete is climbing in the world-renowned Ouray Ice Park. She is at the bottom of the gorge carrying a heavy pack filled with ice-climbing gear. Suddenly, a shelf of ice fractures beneath her feet and the crampons on her right boot twist at an awkward angle. She feels a sharp pain in the lower leg as she falls. When she tries to stand, her leg gives way and will not support her weight.

She very calmly says to a member of the climbing group, "Can you help me? I've broken my leg." The rescuer replies, "There's no way. You would be in so much pain." She asks him to splint her lower extremity with ice tools. When this has been accomplished, she climbs backwards up a 100-foot exit ladder and hobbles with assistance to a car waiting to take her to the emergency department. The hospital evaluation reveals fractures of the tibia and fibula, as well as a completely dislocated foot. She is taken to surgery that evening, where multiple screws and plates are inserted to repair the fractures and dislocation.

The takeaway here is that completely accurate field diagnoses can be difficult for some individuals due to an extreme range of pain tolerance.

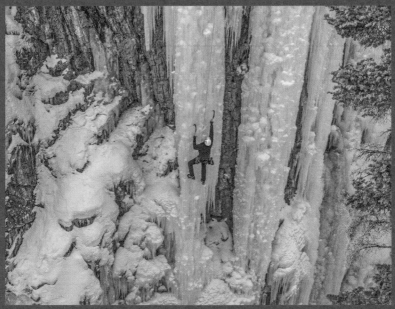

Ouray Ice Park in Colorado

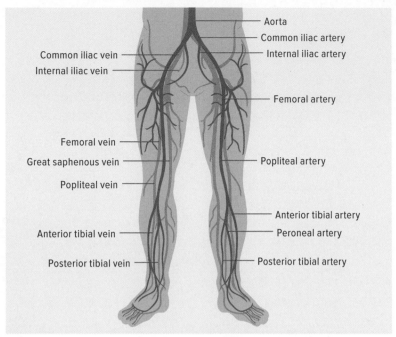

The veins (blue) and arteries (red) of the legs

VASCULAR INJURIES OF THE LOWER EXTREMITIES

The vascular anatomy of the leg is very similar to that of the arm. The vessels are obviously larger because there is more tissue to supply with oxygenated blood in the leg as compared to the arm. The detailed arterial and venous anatomy is shown in the image above.

The names of the specific vessels are not particularly important. The point to remember is that the vessels of the leg are significantly larger than their upper extremity counterparts, which in turn leads to a significantly faster rate of blood loss when injured. Again, the vessels become larger the closer they get to the torso. Any injuries to these large-diameter structures require that definitive treatment be initiated immediately to ensure that the patient does not bleed to death.

To illustrate this point, here is an exercise to try: the large artery in an adult leg is roughly the same diameter as a typical water bladder hose. As discussed previously, when the average adult loses 2 quarts of blood, the chance of survival approaches zero. To give a visual demonstration of how long it takes for a patient to bleed to death after a total transection of the large leg artery (femoral artery), fill a water bladder with 2 quarts of water, take the end cap off the hose, and forcefully squeeze the water out. This squeezing pressure roughly mimics the pressure inside this large artery.

How long did it take to empty the bladder? Roughly a minute. This illustrates the urgency of the situation.

As we progress farther down the leg, the large artery splits at the knee—this time into three arteries, not two as for the arm. Again, transection of these smaller arteries will result in proportionally less blood loss, but it can still represent a life-threatening situation.

As the arteries become progressively smaller in the foot, the bleeding risk diminishes.

The treatment for bleeding injuries and open wounds remains the same as for upper extremity trauma. The first step is to stop the bleeding by direct pressure, pressure points, and/or tourniquets as appropriate. Gently cleaning open wounds and covering them with a clean gauze or cloth is also recommended.

DISLOCATIONS

To allow for movement of the different segments of the extremities, the connecting joints between these segments must pivot so that specific movements or articulations may occur. The majority of joints are called **ball and socket joints.** The anatomic specifics include a rounded end of the

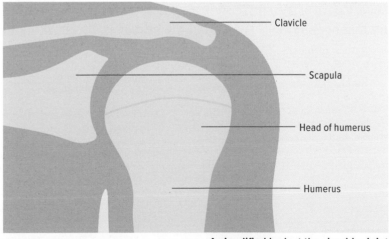

Clavicle

Scapula

Head of humerus

Humerus

A simplified look at the shoulder joint

bone immediately next to the joint, which fits into a concavity in the end of the bone immediately proximal to the joint. The entire joint is then stabilized by strong connective bands called ligaments, which surround the joint. An example of such a joint is the shoulder joint, shown on the previous page.

External trauma that forces the distal rounded bones out of the socket of the proximal bones results in a dislocation of the joint. The socket or cup of the proximal bone, along with the supporting ligaments, are frequently broken or torn in the process. Specific upper extremity dislocations are discussed below.

Shoulder Dislocations

After finger dislocations, shoulders represent the most frequently dislocated joint in the body. This is largely due to the extreme range of motion in the joint. From a geometric standpoint, this hypermobility comes at the expense of stability of the joint. The cup of the proximal bone (scapula) is shallower and the supporting ligaments longer and more flexible. While allowing the upper extremity a rather astounding ability to move in multiple directions, injudicious movements of relatively minor falls on an outstretched arm may dislocate the humerus from the scapula.

About 90% of shoulder dislocations are called **anterior dislocations,** where the head (ball) of the bone slides in front of the socket.

Patients who have suffered such a dislocation will have severe pain of the entire shoulder area with a marked inability to move the arm. The ball of the humerus may be felt and

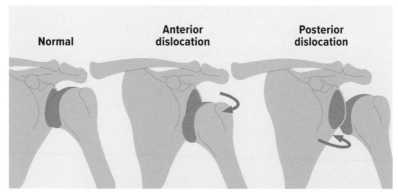

Normal shoulder anatomy and two types of shoulder dislocations

sometimes seen below the level of where it is usually located. A hollow divot is frequently apparent above the now dislocated humerus, especially in lean individuals.

Treatment of shoulder dislocations should be done on a case-by-case basis. Often, patients have experienced multiple dislocations in the past of the same joint and know how to relocate it themselves. If this is the first dislocation episode, this will not be the case.

If help is relatively close by, within a couple of hours, strongly consider placing the affected extremity in a sling and seeking definitive medical care. If this is not the case, the patient and rescuer must decide if they want to try field relocation. Keep in mind that spasm of the surrounding musculature and swelling of the soft tissues will make relocation of the humerus quite difficult. Also consider several key points before making this decision.

First, the inciting trauma may have produced a fracture of the cup of the scapula, and forcing the humerus back into position may worsen the fracture. Second, without the administration of muscle relaxants and pain medications, repositioning the humerus can be extremely difficult, if not impossible. This is especially true for very muscular young men.

Having taken into account these considerations, either a protracted extraction or intolerable pain may warrant a relocation attempt. Two methods are described below.

Shoulder Relocation Method 1   This method works best with two rescuers. With the patient seated, one rescuer holds the patient in place either with their hands or by holding onto a jacket or sleeping bag wrapped around the victim's torso. The second rescuer will kneel close to the patient with their right hand holding the upper arm of the patient in the case of a right-arm dislocation. The rescuer's left hand will firmly grasp the patient's forearm. Then, in a coordinated fashion, the rescuer's right hand will pull outward and downward on the upper arm of the patient while the left hand twists the forearm away from the patient (external rotation).

This will likely be excruciatingly painful for the victim, so pain medication such as ibuprofen or other, stronger medication (only

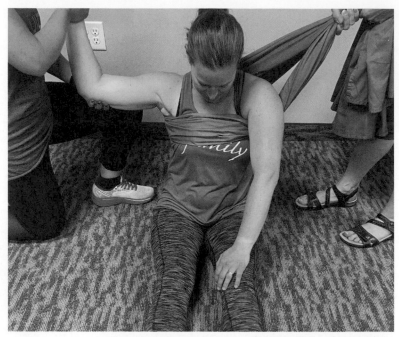

Shoulder relocation method 1

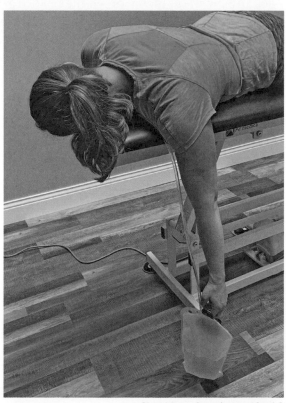

Shoulder relocation method 2

as directed and prescribed by a licensed healthcare provider) administered 30 minutes or so before the relocation attempt may be helpful. This step should be done immediately after the decision to relocate is made so that the medication has time to work.

If the attempt is successful, the head of the humerus (ball) will visibly slide back into place and the patient should experience an immediate sense of pain relief. Very carefully, stabilize the shoulder in a sling, then seek immediate medical care.

If this attempt is unsuccessful, the parties should discuss whether repeated attempts with potential change of rescuer, positioning, and other factors should be considered.

Shoulder Relocation Method 2   A second method that may be used to relocate the shoulder also begins with a considered discussion with the patient followed by the administration of pain medications. As always, medications should only be taken as directed on the label or by a prescribing provider. After enough time has passed to allow the medication to take effect, the patient lays face down on a hard surface such as a log, large rock, or picnic table. The patient must be high enough off the ground so that the extended arm is several feet off the ground. The affected arm is then allowed to dangle freely toward the ground. Next, one or more water bladders are taped to the patient's wrist. Care must be taken to not cut off the circulation to the hand by taping it too tightly. The final step is to slowly fill the water bladders with water. This will apply gradually increasing pressure to the dislocated humerus. As it is pulled downward and away from the cup of the scapula (distracted in medical terms), the ball of the humerus will hopefully clear the edge of the receiving cup. When this happens, the strong shoulder muscles may pull the bone back into its normal position. Additional bladders may be added as needed.

Note: Extreme attempts at relocation should be avoided. The reason for this is that, even if a fracture of one or more bones has not occurred with the initial traumatic insult, inappropriately aggressive relocation attempts may actually break the head of the humerus and/or the cup of the scapula.

POSTERIOR SHOULDER DISLOCATIONS

This situation occurs when the head of the humerus dislocates from the scapular cup and retracts behind or posterior to its normal position. These types of injuries account for less than 10% of all shoulder dislocations.

If you encounter this situation, stabilize the arm in the position of maximum comfort (or minimum discomfort) and initiate rapid evacuation. It is extremely difficult to relocate a posterior shoulder dislocation. This usually must be done in the emergency department or even the operating room.

Elbow Dislocations

In contrast to shoulder dislocations, elbow dislocations occur infrequently and are typically the result of significantly greater external traumatic forces. In the backcountry, elbow dislocations often occur after falls from heights as opposed to falls from a standing position. Children are also more commonly affected by this particular joint dislocation due to their proportionally diminished muscle mass and hypermobility around the elbow joint.

These injuries happen when the forearm is driven forcefully in the general direction of the upper arm while the elbow is bent. This forces the large forearm bone behind the cup at the end of the humerus (see image below).

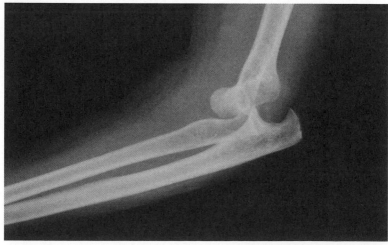

A dislocated elbow on an X-ray

Because of the lack of flexibility of this joint, with the exception of a flexion movement (like a biceps curl motion), these dislocations usually produce fractures of one or more of the bones involved, along with a rupture of the supporting ligaments. For these reasons, relocation of these injuries should not be attempted in the field. Repair in the operating room is frequently required.

The patient's arm should be placed in a sling and stabilized in this position. Ice and ibuprofen are helpful adjuncts to help with pain and swelling.

Wrist Dislocations

Although uncommon, the hand (all or portions thereof) may actually dislocate from the eight small wrist bones (carpal bones) that separate the finger bones (metacarpal bones)

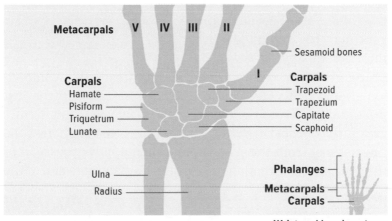

Wrist and hand anatomy

from the two forearm bones (radius and ulna). Similarly, those eight small wrist bones may pop out of the sockets at the end of the forearm bones, resulting in a dislocation of the entire wrist and hand. The normal anatomy is shown above.

Just like the elbow joint, the wrist is held together tightly with strong surrounding ligaments. Forces large enough to dislocate the wrist will usually rupture these ligaments and break the fragile wrist and forearm bones. Again, attempts at field relocation are not advised for these injuries. Splinting the wrist and placing the arm in a sling until definitive medical care can be reached is the standard treatment.

Finger Dislocations

As discussed in the section on finger fractures (pages 155–156), there are multiple joints between the small finger bones. Any of these may dislocate even with relatively minor forces if applied just the right way. Typically, finger dislocations may occur after falling on an outstretched hand with the fingers extended, or while attempting to catch a forcefully thrown ball. While painful and unsightly (see right), finger dislocations do not generally represent a serious injury.

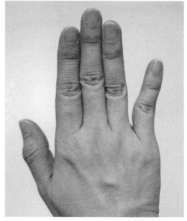

A dislocated finger

Unlike the two previously mentioned dislocations, field relocation of dislocated fingers may be attempted with little accompanying risk. The procedure to do so is relatively straightforward. A companion simply holds the portion of the dislocated finger just proximal (closest to the heart) to the dislocated joint, firmly grasps the dislocated distal portion, pulls that portion of the finger away from the patient, and then applies pressure in the appropriate direction to relocate the dislocated end of the

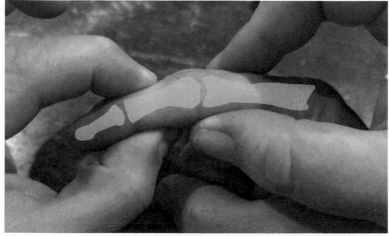

A simple guide to field treatment of a dislocated finger

finger back into line with the portion of the digit closest to the wrist.

Although it is possible that a bone may be chipped in the relocation process, this is not likely and not terribly clinically significant even if it does occur. The relief that the patient will feel is usually immediate and profound.

Bear in mind that the injured digit will swell, so if you choose to tape it to an adjacent finger for protection, it must be done with a loose and/or noncircumferential wrap to avoid compromising the blood supply to the finger.

It is generally advisable to obtain an X-ray of the hand when the patient arrives back in civilization to make sure there is no fracture to the finger.

SOFT TISSUE INJURIES AND BLEEDING

Since humans typically use their extremities to interact with the environment, these frontline appendages see more than their fair share of injuries. Aside from fractures and dislocations, the soft tissues (skin, muscles, nerves, and blood vessels) are at risk for all sorts of mayhem in the back-country, including bruising, crush injuries, lacerations, and even amputations. Soft tissue extremity injuries are broadly divided into two categories: those that breach the skin integrity and those where the skin remains intact.

Soft tissue trauma that does not result in a fracture and/or dislocation most commonly causes only bruising. Although such bruising may be quite painful and ugly with black/blue/yellow discoloration, these sorts of traumatic events do not usually provoke significant clinical concern. Treatment includes ice, ibuprofen, and elevation if possible.

More severe traumatic events that result in tearing or laceration of the skin and/or underlying tissue may be more dangerous due to blood loss and infection considerations. In the backcountry, in circumstances where the extraction of an individual may take days, blood loss represents the more pressing concern.

To better understand how to treat severe blood loss due to an upper extremity injury, we must first understand the anatomy of the blood vessels.

As described in previous chapters, the vascular system consists of two discrete systems. The first consists of arteries that distribute oxygenated, fresh blood from the heart to all of the tissues in the body. This includes organs, muscles, bones, and skin. The second phase of blood circulation consists of veins, or the venous system. The veins collect the now oxygen-depleted, toxin-laden blood from the tissues and transport it back to the heart where it is pumped through the lungs to be cleansed and reoxygenated once again.

The difference between these two sets of hollow transport tubes is as follows:

Arteries

- Have thick, muscular walls that possess the capacity to forcefully expand and contract to maintain the appropriate blood pressure
- May contract aggressively if injured in an attempt to limit blood loss
- See the same high, pulsatile pressures as the heart (ideally 120/80 mm/Hg)
- Become progressively smaller after they exit the heart

Veins

- Have very thin walls without the ability to expand and contract
- Cannot constrict when injured to stem blood loss
- See very low, non-pulsatile pressures (8–12 mm/Hg)
- Become progressively larger as they approach the heart

Obviously, the larger the blood vessel, either artery or vein, the greater the potential for significant blood loss in the event of an injury. In other words, the closer to the heart, the larger the diameter of the artery or vein, and thus the higher the risk to the life of the patient if the wall of the vessel is breached.

Having said that, as the vessels become larger, they are also tucked in close to an overlying large bone. This means that if an injury occurs to the vessel, it may be compressed against the protecting bone by the hands of a rescuer to help stop the bleeding. This method of compressing the site of bleeding is known as direct pressure and should be the very first maneuver tried to staunch significant bleeding.

An example of how this works would be an injury to the largest artery in the arm—the brachial artery—which courses inside the humerus. Any injury here could lead to a fatal hemorrhage in just a few minutes. To stop this, a rescuer would use both hands to squeeze shut the injured artery. Specifically, the rescuer would place both thumbs on the outer part of the upper arm, encircle the arm on either side, and use the fingers to compress the injured artery against the humerus, thus shutting off the flow.

Obviously, such a situation represents a true emergency, and the most expeditious evacuation method should be taken while the rescuer is holding pressure.

For prolonged extractions, or in situations where the rescuer cannot stem the flow, a tourniquet may be applied. As described previously, this should only be placed in true life-threatening situations where there is no other option. A tourniquet will completely shut off the flow of oxygenated blood to the extremity. The limb will suffer irreversible ischemia (lack of blood flow) within only a few hours.

As we progress farther down the arm into the forearm, the arteries split into smaller-in-diameter ones. When transected, these smaller arteries bleed less than the larger ones, but they can still represent a threat to the patient's life if they are allowed to bleed without intervention.

At the elbow, the single large brachial artery divides into two arteries: the radial artery and the ulnar artery. These vessels run along with their correspondingly named bones for protection. Again, damage to these arteries requires a rescuer to compress them with one or both hands against the bony "backboard" to stop the bleeding. Tourniquets are much less frequently required in this location but may occasionally be necessary depending on rescuer availability, time to definitive medical care, additional injuries, and other problems.

Arterial injuries distal to the wrist (i.e., fingers) will either stop on their own accord or be able to be closed with finger compression either by the patient or a rescuer. A tourniquet is almost never required for these injuries.

Injuries to veins may always be treated with simple, direct pressure due to their extremely low pressure. Tourniquets are essentially never warranted for these injuries.

To review, arterial bleeding is recognized as being bright red and pulsatile, while venous bleeding manifests as dark, non-pulsatile or oozing. Certainly, injuries to both arteries and veins may be present especially for more significant traumatic events.

Pressure Points

Although not commonly required, compressing a damaged vessel near the site of injury may be a useful adjunct to direct pressure. This may be required if direct pressure does not

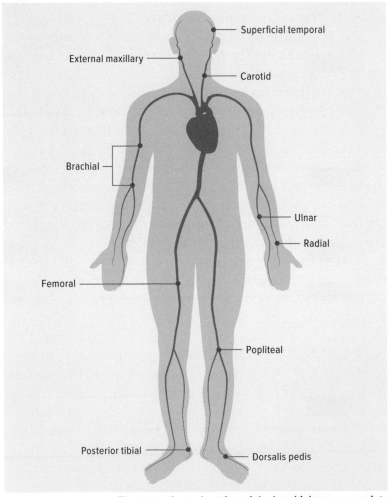

The approximate location of the brachial pressure points

stop the bleeding or the site of injury is not readily accessible for some reason.

For the upper extremity, the armpit may be forcefully compressed in the situation where a brachial artery injury is encountered and cannot be controlled with direct pressure. This maneuver can be continued while a tourniquet is being prepared.

For arterial injuries of the forearm and beyond, the brachial artery may be compressed against the distal humerus next to the elbow joint. As opposed to the armpit, this site is much easier to access and manage a complete closure of the vessel.

Lacerations and Avulsions

When a sharp object cuts through the skin and underlying tissues, a **laceration** results. The primary treatment objective is to staunch any bleeding as described above. After this has been accomplished, the wound may be gently cleaned and dressed. To clean any open wound in the field, simply pour some clean water over the injury to remove any gross contamination, and then loosely wrap a clean gauze or cloth around the site. Do not attempt to forcefully instill water or poke about inside the wound. This has the potential to drive foreign objects farther into the soft tissues.

When a portion of the skin and/or underlying soft tissues has been completely ripped away, an **avulsion** has occurred. Treatment remains the same as for lacerations: stop the bleeding, gently cleanse the wound if appropriate, and wrap loosely with a clean cloth or gauze.

HOW TO REMOVE AN EMBEDDED FISHHOOK

Most people who enjoy fishing will have either a personal account of a fishhook embedded in some body part, or they will know someone who has suffered such an event. The rearward-facing barb on the hook that makes it so effective in capturing a fish will also make it

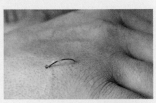

An embedded fishhook, a common outdoor injury

essentially impossible to remove by pulling it out backwards. This can, of course, be attempted, especially if it has not penetrated very far into the underlying tissue.

More than likely, however, a more involved extraction process will be needed. One of two distinct methods will likely be required to remove the hook. Both will be much more pleasant for the patient if a local, injectable anesthetic (such as lidocaine) is available for use by qualified medical personnel. The local anesthetic may be injected under sterile conditions at the site of entry of the hook. The removal can also be done without the use of a local anesthetic, but this is not recommended. A small incision may be made at the site. The tissues are then spread with a hemostat or similar tool, and the hook is pulled backwards.

The second method becomes useful when the hook has embedded deeply into the tissue and the point of the hook has lodged just below the skin level. The area over the point may be injected with local anesthetic. The incision is made at this point and the hook is pushed forward and out. If need be, the hook may be cut with a pair of wire cutters to facilitate removal.

Ideally, the patient should be transported to the nearest emergency room, where the hook can be removed by a qualified physician under more controlled conditions.

If the removal is performed in the backcountry, the wound must be washed with clean water and covered with a clean bandage. Watch for signs of infection, such as increasing redness at the penetration site, purulent discharge, or fever.

BURNS AND ELECTRICAL ACCIDENTS

Burns represent a special category in the trauma lexicon. Although not nearly as common in the backcountry as in the confined spaces of urban settings, severe burns that occur far from advanced medical care represent a true emergency.

As with all medical and trauma considerations, prevention is key for these very serious and potentially life-altering or even life-ending injuries. Fire safety should always be high on our safety checklist, not only to prevent injuries to ourselves and our companions, but also to protect our precious environment.

You should only build a campfire when it's allowed by the National Forest Service or other governing body. Additionally, you should only build a fire in existing sites. Campfires should be small, and all fuel sources, such as dry grass, overhanging limbs, etc., should be cleared. It is also important to just use common sense. If fires are officially permitted, but the local conditions such as wind, dry fuel sources, etc., are present, skip the fire altogether.

All campfires should be "dead out" upon leaving the site. Dousing the site with water, stirring it with a stick to soak all buried hot coals, and adding a final layer of dirt are imperative steps to ensure the safety of our national treasures.

Camp stoves represent the other potential source of burn injury. Never use a stove inside a tent due to the potential for carbon monoxide poisoning along with the potential fire hazard. Nylon tents burn very quickly and very hot.

Burns are characterized based on depth of injury, location, and surface area involved. Burn depth is described as follows.

First degree   Sunburn (see page 27)

Second degree   Also called partial thickness burns, these burns destroy the skin layers up to but not including the layer immediately under the superficial skin layers (epidermis). This underlayer is called the dermis and appears as a white, shiny surface when exposed. Second-degree burns are often further subcategorized into superficial and deep, depending on depth of penetration. These burns are quite painful.

Third degree   These injuries extend all the way through the epidermal and dermal layers and into the subcutaneous fat layers. Paradoxically, these burns are not painful to the touch because the superficial sensory nerves of the skin have been destroyed by the burning process.

Fourth degree   These injuries are associated with high-voltage electrical injuries such as lightning strikes and touching high-voltage electrical wires.

Burn injuries either occur by thermal events or by direct contact of caustic material such as acids or alkalis (corrosive substances). Thermal burns are much more common and, in the backcountry, usually are the result of campfire or stove

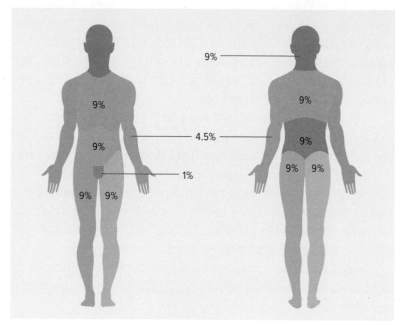

Diagram 1

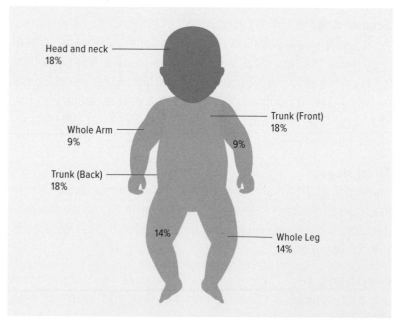

Diagram 2

accidents. The first order of business in terms of treatment consists of removing the burning material, including clothes, from the individual. Time is obviously of the essence here, so the rescuer must act immediately. If the victim's clothes are still on fire, they can be rolled in the dirt, or, if available, pour a container of water on the area.

After the burning material is extinguished, the burned area may be briefly rinsed with water only. The burned area should then be *loosely* covered with a clean dressing. We strongly emphasize loosely because burned tissue swells so vigorously that it is difficult to imagine the final size of the burned part unless you have experienced such an episode. Tight wraps around a burned extremity, for instance, can result in compromise of blood flow to the tissue distal to the bandage. This may easily and quickly result in amputation of the extremity beyond this point.

Immediate medical care should be sought for all but the smallest burns, especially those burns involving the face, hands, or genitalia.

The amount of surface area of burned skin is also critical when assessing the severity of the injury. Diagrams 1 and 2 on the facing page demonstrate how to estimate burn size so that the rescuers may relay this information to the burn care team.

Young children and infants have proportionately larger heads, and their TBSA (Total Body Surface Area) burn estimation is shown in Diagram 2. Note the comparison to the adult TBSA estimation.

Should there be a delay in evacuating severely burned individuals, two considerations become evident very quickly. First, burned tissue weeps a tremendous amount of fluid. If these fluids are not replaced quickly and aggressively, the patient may die from fluid and electrolyte loss. In the burn units of trauma centers, the individuals may receive 10 liters or more of intravenous electrolyte solutions per day. Until definitive evacuation is completed, the patient must take in copious amounts of water and electrolytes by mouth if they are able. The amount of fluids given can be determined by the patient's urine output. "Clear and copious" is the catch-phrase here. It should be emphasized that these fluid losses are ongoing and must therefore be continuously replaced.

The second consideration is infection. Burn wounds can allow the ingress of bacteria and other pathogens due to the loss of integrity of the skin as a barrier to these pathogens. Such infections can overwhelm the body's defense mechanisms in a very short time. If a patient is not able to receive definitive medical attention quickly, and signs and symptoms of infection manifest, consider administering whatever antibiotics are available by mouth. Infectious indications include fever, redness and/or pus at the wound areas, tachycardia (elevated heart rate), confusion, and drop in blood pressure.

Fourth-degree burns merit special mention for several reasons. First, the energy transfer from either a high-voltage power line or a lightning strike is tremendous. By definition, a significant amount of that energy will be transferred to the tissues in the path of the electric current. For such injuries, there will always be a relatively small entrance wound and a much larger exit wound. All tissue between these two sites is at risk for complete destruction. This even includes bone. That defines fourth-degree burns—destruction of the deepest muscles/organs/bones in the body.

The electric current will often cause cardiac arrest, so bystanders should assess for pulses and start CPR and acquire an AED immediately.

It goes without saying that, with or without cardiac arrest, all patients who survive such incidents must be evacuated to the nearest hospital immediately.

LIGHTNING

As mentioned above, the most immediately negative consequence of a lightning injury short of death is cardiac arrest. If this occurs, bystanders should immediately begin CPR as instructed previously.

As with all injuries, the most important treatment component of lightning injuries is prevention. Consider these steps whenever venturing into the backcountry, where lightning events are common.

- First, examine weather conditions for your proposed travel destinations and for the duration of your trip. Multiple good apps are available for smartphones for this purpose. The National Weather Service information is always a good place to start.

- Make sure you understand the typical characteristics of electric storm cells. Thunderheads (electrically charged storm clouds) discharge pent-up electricity via cloud-to-ground strikes. These discharges usually hit the tallest object in the area. This is common but by no means universal. If you're caught in such a storm, it is essential to not seek shelter under an isolated tree or small stand of trees.

- Water conducts electric currents beautifully. Therefore, it is imperative to not perch on top of rocks. They will be wet from the accompanying rain, and even if a person is not directly struck by a bolt, a nearby strike may conduct the current via the wet rocks and result in serious or even fatal injuries.

- Finally, metal is an extremely good conductor of electricity. You should remove all metal objects from packs, pockets, etc.

It is impossible to outrun a thunderstorm. If you happen to be above tree line, however, it is prudent to move downhill and into a heavily forested area.

If you must weather such a storm, the proper positioning is crouched either on top of bare ground or a pack with no metal. Take care to stay away from objective hazards such as cliffs. There have been reports of indirect lightning strikes bouncing people off cliffs.

EMERGENCY KITS AND OTHER HELPFUL GEAR

It makes good sense, especially when traveling into the backcountry, to keep complete medical and emergency preparedness kits in the vehicle. A hard case is ideal for such kits. These items will come in handy for two distinct scenarios. First, if you're venturing far afield, some mechanical malfunction may occur to the transport vehicle. Help may be difficult to obtain due to lack of cell reception, lack of time involved in accessing a remote location, or lack of emergency response personnel. For this reason, backcountry travelers should keep with them the means to survive for at least several days, if not longer. These survival pieces of equipment are divided into medical and emergency preparedness kits.

Car Medical Kit

- ALL medications for each member of the party for at least a week
- Additional medications
- Ibuprofen
- Tylenol
- EpiPen, Children's EpiPen
- Ciprofloxacin
- Bactrim
- Metronidazole
- Cortisone cream
- Eye drops/antibiotic eye drops
- Electrolyte tabs/powder or premixed drink
- Antinausea medication, such as Phenergan tablets/ suppositories, Zofran sublingual tablet

- Bandages, including gauze, coband (stretchy wrap), adhesive bandages of various sizes
- Athletic tape
- Steri-Strips and benzoin (to make strips stick to skin)
- Chemical heat/cold packs

Car Emergency Kit

- Sleeping bags/pads
- Flares/chem-lights/flashlights
- Several days rations of food and water for each member of the party
- Emergency shelter (tent, bivvy sack)
- Spare clothing, especially in cold weather
- Phone battery backup chargers or solar chargers
- Air compressor
- Ropes/tie downs
- Extra fuel, antifreeze, washer fluid, and motor oil

Backcountry Expedition Kit

It becomes extremely difficult to configure a single backcountry expedition medical kit that will be ideal for every remote adventure. The size and contents of the kit will vary greatly depending on the underlying medical conditions of the team members, the objective, the remoteness, and other factors. All equipment lists in the backcountry represent some sort of compromise. Weight is often viewed as a more important consideration than taking medical supplies to cover every possible exigency, for instance. To this end, we will outline supplies that would be ideal to take. You will have to pick and choose depending on your particular objective.

- Medications
- Ibuprofen (200 mg)
- Tylenol (500 mg)
- Zofran sublingual tabs (4 mg)
- Phenergan suppositories (25 mg)

- Phenergan tablets (25 mg)
- Acetazolamide (for acclimatization only—250 mg; recommend ½ tab in AM only)
- Antihistamine (Benadryl)
- Dexamethasone (tablets and injections)
- Ciprofloxacin (500 mg)
- Metronidazole (500 mg)
- Bactrim (100 mg)
- Antibiotic eye drops
- Adult and children's EpiPens
- Dental paste to repair broken teeth, lost fillings, and crowns
- Bandages—self-adhesive, various sizes; gauze; self-adherent wrap (coband, vet wrap, etc.)
- Elastic wraps
- Athletic/duct tape
- Steri-Strips
- Benzoin spray or liquid pop tubes (to make Steri-Strips adhere to skin)
- Oxygen bottles, nasal cannula, face mask
- Gamow bag

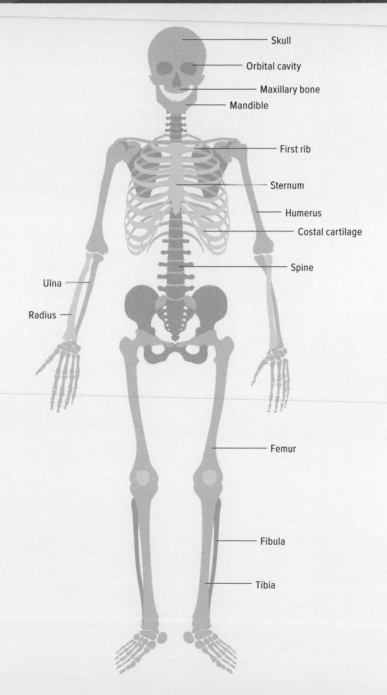

Skull

Orbital cavity

Maxillary bone

Mandible

First rib

Sternum

Humerus

Costal cartilage

Spine

Ulna

Radius

Femur

Fibula

Tibia

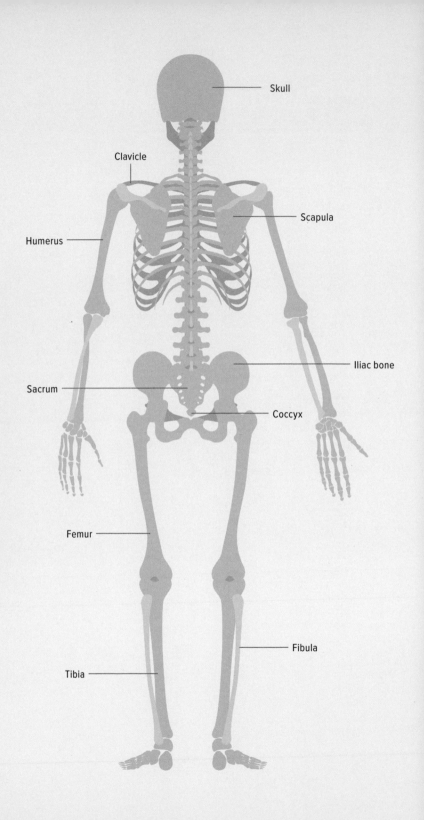

Skull

Clavicle

Scapula

Humerus

Iliac bone

Sacrum

Coccyx

Femur

Fibula

Tibia

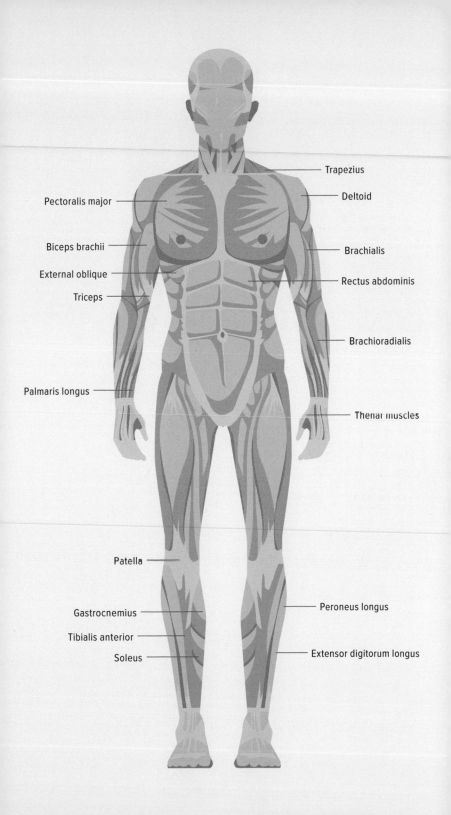

Trapezius

Pectoralis major

Deltoid

Biceps brachii

Brachialis

External oblique

Rectus abdominis

Triceps

Brachioradialis

Palmaris longus

Thenar muscles

Patella

Gastrocnemius

Peroneus longus

Tibialis anterior

Soleus

Extensor digitorum longus

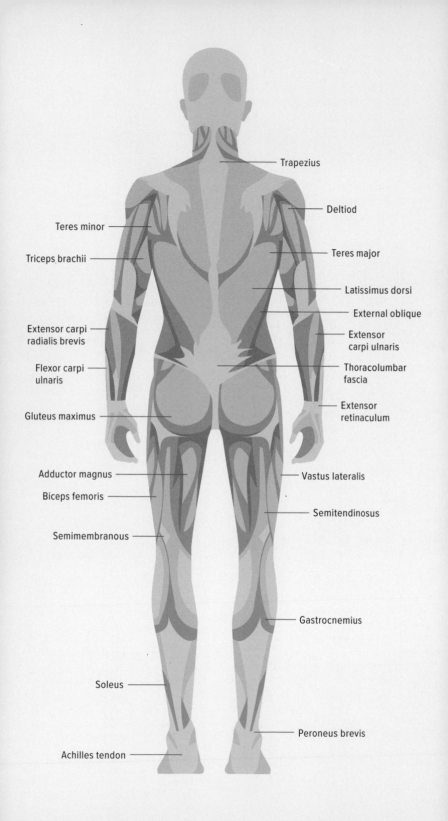

Trapezius

Deltiod

Teres minor

Teres major

Triceps brachii

Latissimus dorsi

External oblique

Extensor carpi
radialis brevis

Extensor
carpi ulnaris

Flexor carpi
ulnaris

Thoracolumbar
fascia

Gluteus maximus

Extensor
retinaculum

Adductor magnus

Vastus lateralis

Biceps femoris

Semitendinosus

Semimembranous

Gastrocnemius

Soleus

Peroneus brevis

Achilles tendon

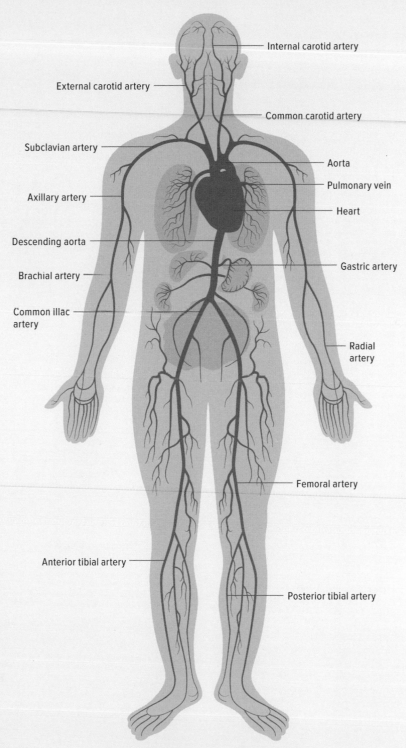

Internal carotid artery

External carotid artery

Common carotid artery

Subclavian artery

Aorta

Pulmonary vein

Axillary artery

Heart

Descending aorta

Gastric artery

Brachial artery

Common illac artery

Radial artery

Femoral artery

Anterior tibial artery

Posterior tibial artery

Arterial view of the human circulatory system

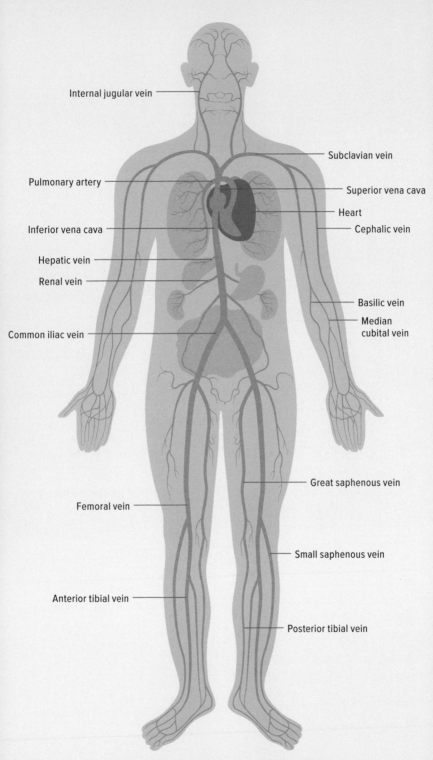

Internal jugular vein

Subclavian vein

Pulmonary artery

Superior vena cava

Heart

Inferior vena cava

Cephalic vein

Hepatic vein

Renal vein

Basilic vein

Median cubital vein

Common iliac vein

Great saphenous vein

Femoral vein

Small saphenous vein

Anterior tibial vein

Posterior tibial vein

Venous view of the human circulatory system

RECOMMENDED RESOURCES

WEBSITES

Cleveland Clinic Health Library
my.clevelandclinic.org/health

Mayo Clinic
mayoclinic.org/patient-care-and-health-information

Merck Manual, Home Edition (free)
merckmanuals.com/home

RECOMMENDED READING

DK. *American College of Emergency Physicians First Aid Manual: The Step-by-Step Guide for Everyone* (5th ed.). London: DK Publishing (Dorling Kindersley), 2014.

Roberts, A. *The Complete Human Body: The Definitive Visual Guide* (2nd ed.). London: DK Publishing (Dorling Kindersley), 2016.

Schimelpfenig, T. *NOLS Wilderness Medicine* (7th ed.). Mechanicsburg, PA: Stackpole Books, 2021.

FIRST AID, CPR, AND WILDERNESS MEDICINE COURSES

American Red Cross
redcross.org/take-a-class

NOLS Wilderness Medicine
nols.edu/en/wilderness-medicine/courses/get-certified

Wilderness Medicine Training Center
wildmedcenter.com

QUICK REFERENCE INDEX

INDEX

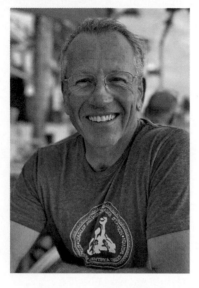

Patrick Brighton is a board-certified general and trauma surgeon who lives high in the mountains of Colorado. Along with his wife, he has been fortunate to travel extensively and experience the wonders of the remote areas of our planet. From adventure racing in the unexplored jungles of Borneo to traversing the high peaks of the Andes to scaling Himalayan peaks, he has practiced a wide range of outdoor sports.

He is currently the captain of the Ouray Mountain Rescue Team in southwest Colorado and counts himself fortunate to be surrounded by some of the world's leading experts in the realm of mountain rescue.

He has extensive experience in caring for trauma victims, including the management of multiple mass-casualty events, as well as providing care to patients in the line of duty as a rescue team member. This unique knowledge base allows him to impart wilderness medicine information from the perspective of someone who has been responsible for the complete care of injured individuals, from the time of injury to the diagnostic and therapeutic phases to rehabilitation. This rich experience forms the foundation of the practical and easy-to-understand information presented in this book.